ABC of
Tubes, Drains, Lines and Frames

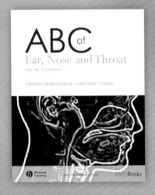
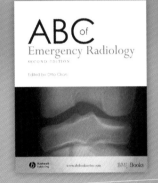
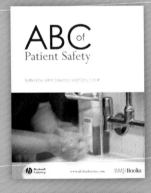
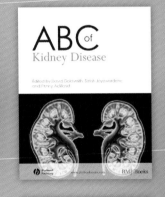
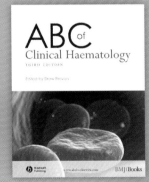
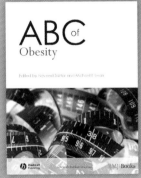

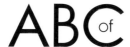

ABC of

Tubes, Drains, Lines and Frames

EDITED BY

Adam Brooks

Consultant in HPB & Emergency Surgery
Nottingham University NHS Trust
Nottingham, UK and
Senior Lecturer in Military Surgery and Trauma
The Royal Centre for Defence Medicine
Birmingham, UK

Peter Mahoney

Defence Professor of Anaesthesia and Critical Care
The Royal Centre for Defence Medicine
Birmingham, UK

Brian Rowlands

Professor of Surgery
Nottingham University NHS Trust and
University of Nottingham
Nottingham, UK

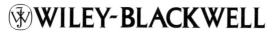

WILEY-BLACKWELL

A John Wiley & Sons, Ltd., Publication

BMJ|Books

This edition first published 2008, © 2008 by Blackwell Publishing Ltd

BMJ Books is an imprint of BMJ Publishing Group Limited, used under licence by Blackwell Publishing which was acquired by John Wiley & Sons in February 2007. Blackwell's publishing programme has been merged with Wiley's global Scientific, Technical and Medical business to form Wiley-Blackwell.

Registered office: John Wiley & Sons Ltd, The Atrium, Southern Gate, Chichester, West Sussex, PO19 8SQ, UK

Editorial offices: 9600 Garsington Road, Oxford, OX4 2DQ, UK
The Atrium, Southern Gate, Chichester, West Sussex, PO19 8SQ, UK
111 River Street, Hoboken, NJ 07030–5774, USA

For details of our global editorial offices, for customer services and for information about how to apply for permission to reuse the copyright material in this book please see our website at www.wiley.com/wiley-blackwell

Library of Congress Cataloging-in-Publication Data

ABC of tubes, drains, lines, and frames / edited by Adam Brooks, Peter Mahoney, Brian Rowlands
p. ; cm.
Includes index.
ISBN: 978-1-4051-6014-8 (alk. paper)
1. Postoperative care--Equipment and supplies. 2. Surgical instruments and apparatus. I. Brooks, Adam, 1969- II. Mahoney, Peter F. III. Rowlands, Brian J.
[DNLM: 1. Postoperative Care--instrumentation--Handbooks. 2. Postoperative Care--methods--Handbooks. 3. Fracture Fixation--instrumentation--Handbooks. 4. Fracture Fixation--methods--Handbooks. 5. Wound Healing--Handbooks. WO 39 A1335 2008]
RD51.A23 2008
617'.919--dc22

2007038359

A catalogue record for this book is available from the British Library.

Set in 9.25/12 pt Minion by Newgen Imaging Systems Pvt. Ltd, Chennai, India
Printed and bound in Singapore by COS Printers Pte Ltd

1   2008

Contents

Contributors

Iain Anderson
Consultant Surgeon, Department of Surgery, Hope Hospital, Salford, Royal NHS Foundation Trust, Manchester, UK

Sherif Awad
Specialist Registrar in General Surgery, Queen's Medical Centre Campus, Nottingham University NHS Trust, Nottingham, UK

Ian Beckingham
Consultant Hepatobiliary Surgeon, Queen's Medical Centre Campus, Nottingham University NHS Trust, Nottingham, UK

Tracy R. Bilski
Assistant Professor of Traumatology and Surgical Critical Care, University of Mississippi Medical Center, Jackson, Mississippi, USA

Adam Brooks
Consultant in HPB & Emergency Surgery, Nottingham University NHS Trust, Nottingham, UK and Senior Lecturer in Military Surgery and Trauma, The Royal Centre for Defence Medicine, Birmingham, UK

Neil Buxton
Consultant Neurosurgeon, Walton Centre for Neurology and Neurosurgery, Alder Hay Hospital, Liverpool, UK

Ben Davies
SpR Cardiothoracic Surgeon, West Midlands Rotation, UK

Joy Field
Clinical Nurse Specialist, Queen's Medical Centre Campus, Nottingham University NHS Trust, Nottingham, UK

J. Edward Fitzgerald
Specialist Registrar and Clinical Teaching Fellow, Medical Education Unit, University of Nottingham Medical School, Nottingham, UK

Dileep Lobo
Associate Professor and Reader in Surgery, Queen's Medical Centre Campus, Nottingham University NHS Trust, Nottingham, UK

Peter Mahoney
Defence Professor of Anaesthesia and Critical Care, The Royal Centre for Defence Medicine, Birmingham, UK

Gurminder Mann
Consultant Urologist, Nottingham City Hospital Campus, Nottingham University NHS Trust, Nottingham, UK

Jonathan Mole
Consultant Anaesthetist, Queen's Medical Centre Campus, Nottingham University NHS Trust, Nottingham, UK

Ian Pallister
Senior Lecturer/Honorary Consultant, Trauma and Orthopaedics, Morrison Hospital, Swansea, UK

Gabriel Rodrigues
Hepatopancreaticobiliary Surgical Fellow, Queen's Medical Centre Campus, Nottingham University NHS Trust, Nottingham, UK

Jerard Ross
Consultant Neurosurgeon, Walton Centre for Neurology and Neurosurgery, Alder Hay Hospital, Liverpool, UK

Brian Rowlands
Professor of Surgery, Queen's Medical Centre Campus, Nottingham University NHS Trust, Nottingham, UK

Alastair Simpson
Specialist Registrar in General Surgery, Queen's Medical Centre Campus, Nottingham University NHS Trust, Nottingham, UK

Amanda Smith
Senior Entero-stomal Therapist Nurse, Hope Hospital, Salford Royal NHS Foundation Trust, Manchester, UK

Andrew Taylor
Consultant in Anaesthesia and Critical Care, Sherwood Forest Hospitals NHS Trust, Foundation Trust, Nottingham, UK

Trudy Towell
Consultant Nurse in Pain Management, Queen's Medical Centre Campus, Nottingham University NHS Trust, Nottingham, UK

Dawn Williams
Advanced Nurse Practitioner in Neurosurgery, Walton Centre for Neurology and Neurosurgery, Alder Hay Hospital, Liverpool, UK

Adam Wolverson
Consultant Anaesthetist, Department of Anaesthetics, Lincoln County Hospital, UK

Preface

Forty years ago when I qualified from Guy's Hospital, the day-to-day activities of medical students and house officers were very different from those of current graduates. As 'surgical dressers' and 'medical ward clerks' we had significant responsibility for a range of patient management tasks that were regarded as essential for the smooth running of the clinical service. Student doctors and nurses learned to dress wounds, keep accurate fluid balance charts and update patient progress notes on a regular basis under the watchful eyes of the ward sister and our immediate seniors. We were participants rather than observers. The skills and knowledge obtained from the regular performance of mundane, but essential tasks, was an important apprenticeship for the acquisition of new skills during specialist professional training. As a surgical trainee in Sheffield I was expected to have an in-depth knowledge of wound care, the management of tubes, stomas and drains, pain control and practical applications of nutritional support. My consultants and senior registrars would ask me to justify any therapeutic decisions, such as the timing of nasogastric tube removal, during ward rounds and teaching sessions. Much of the discussion about 'ward lore' was surgical dogma passed from one generation of trainee to the next. The evidence base was weak and rudimentary. Subsequently, the high dependency and intensive care units introduced new technology and innovations. This strengthened the evidence base and ensured that the most sick patients were monitored more closely using more invasive methods. Experts emerged and developed highly tuned approaches to the care of the critically ill patient. This led to 'de-skilling' of segments of the health care team especially amongst nursing staff, medical students and junior ward staff. They could not easily embrace these advances and were disenfranchised from the continuum of surgical care.

This book is an attempt to restore interest in the evidence base for routine ward care and high dependency care. The germ was the realization that even in the 'high tech' areas there is ignorance and confusion about the principles of good surgical practice such as wound care and stoma management. This has grown into a document that sets out the knowledge, skills and evidence base that underpins good medical care on the surgical wards. The content is basic and practical and will encourage a reawakening of interest in the practical aspects of ward management. Recently, a session on 'Tubes, wounds, stents, stomas and drains' at the Annual Meeting of the Association of the Surgeons of Great Britain and Ireland (ASGBI) in Manchester in April 2007 attracted over 200 participants, the majority of whom were surgical trainees. Their enthusiasm for the topics underscored the necessity for this type of information among trainees. Once the principles of optimal patient management have been embraced, students, nurses and trainees should be encouraged to return to the ward environment to appreciate 'on the job' applications of these simple techniques that improve patient care. Attention to these details should improve outcomes for many patients. Read, learn and enjoy making a difference.

Brian Rowlands

Acknowledgements

We wish to thank the following for their valuable comments on the manuscript and their assistance during the development of the project: Dr Katherine Rice MSc MRCP MRCGP; Mr Andrew Love, Charge Nurse Surgical High Dependency Unit, Queen's Medical Centre; The Staff of the Surgical High Dependency Unit, Queen's Medical Centre, Nottingham; Mr Ed Fitzgerald MRCS.

Adam Brooks
Peter Mahoney
Brian Rowlands

CHAPTER 1

The Complex Abdomen

Tracy R. Bilski, Brian Rowlands and Adam Brooks

OVERVIEW

- Damage control is the staged operative care of the patient to prevent or interrupt the lethal triad of hypothermia, coagulopathy and acidosis
- Initial damage control surgery focuses solely on the control of haemorrhage and contamination
- Temporary abdominal closure techniques are applied if fascial closure is not possible or inadvisable
- Abdominal compartment syndrome is raised intra-abdominal pressure that leads to impaired perfusion of the viscera and systemic sequelae
- The complex abdomen patient requires the coordination of multiple therapies, investigations and interventions over a protracted time

Introduction

The abdomen is a common source of complications in surgical patients (Box 1.1). Perioperative wound problems and issues with abdominal drains can occur as a result of patient disease as well as problems with postoperative care. Treatment of these patients requires meticulous wound and drain care as well as a high index of suspicion for complications. Recent changes to the approach of injured, seriously ill or septic surgical patients has led to an increasing number of patients initially managed with multiple staged procedures and open abdomens. These patients require great commitment from medical and nursing teams, which must span the duration of the hospitalization as well as re-integration and care in the community.

The open abdomen

Definitions

When the abdominal fascia is unable to be re-approximated following laparotomy the result is an *open abdomen*. Typically, this occurs following major trauma and a *damage control* procedure or with intra-abdominal catastrophes and frank abdominal sepsis. The

Box 1.1 **Case study**

A 44-year-old male was involved in a motor vehicle crash sustaining injuries to the colon and a laceration to the spleen. At laparotomy he underwent resection and anastomosis of the colon and a splenectomy. On postoperative day 8 he spiked a fever with a discharge from the lower aspect of his wound. Later that day the surgeon was urgently called as bowel was clearly protruding through the skin. The bowel was covered with saline-soaked gauze and the patient urgently taken to the operating room where a complete breakdown of the anastomosis with free pus and faecal spillage was discovered. He underwent an abdominal washout and diversion procedure (end colostomy) with a VAC dressing and the placement of two tube drains. His critical care course was very unstable and involved numerous abdominal procedures to control sepsis. Eventually a Vicryl™ mesh was placed over the bowel and allowed to granulate before the placement of a split thickness skin graft. He was finally discharged home 45 days after his initial injuries requiring continuing wound care to his skin-grafted abdomen and an abdominal binder to support his large abdominal hernia.

open abdomen may also be a result of a *decompressive laparotomy* for *abdominal compartment syndrome* (ACS) (Figure 1.1).

Damage control is the staged operative care of the patient to prevent or interrupt the lethal triad of hypothermia, coagulopathy and acidosis. *Damage control surgery* for the abdomen refers to an abbreviated laparotomy for trauma or emergency surgery that focuses solely on the control of hemorrhage and contamination (Figure 1.2). There are three phases:
- *Phase I*. Control of hemorrhage and contamination – definitive reconstruction is delayed. Temporary abdominal dressing or skin closure performed.
- *Phase II*. Restoration of physiology in the intensive care unit (ICU).
- *Phase III*. Re-operation for removal of packing, definitive repair of injury and closure if possible. At this stage fascial closure may not be possible.

Reasons for leaving the abdomen open
- In trauma or emergency surgery, unstable physiology necessitating a truncated laparotomy with expedited move of the patient to the ICU for correction of physiological derangement.

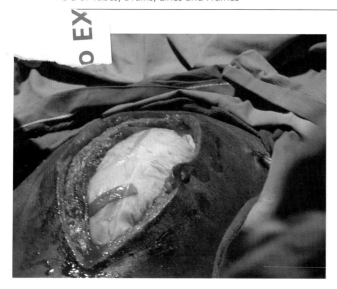

Figure 1.1 Patient with an open abdomen.

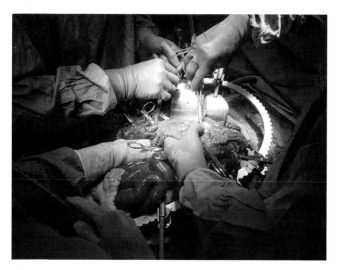

Figure 1.2 Damage control surgery.

- In other surgical procedures where the patient develops similar unstable physiology (e.g. ruptured abdominal aorta, acute mesenteric ischaemia).
- Oedematous bowel unable to be fully reduced into the abdomen without causing signs/symptoms of *intra-abdominal hypertension* or *ACS*.
- In gross abdominal sepsis from bowel perforation or anastomotic breakdown.
- Abdominal compartment syndrome.

Intra-abdominal hypertension refers to elevated intra-abdominal pressure (normal 5–7 mmHg).

Abdominal compartment syndrome

- Clinical scenario whereby intra-abdominal hypertension results in impaired perfusion of the viscera and systemic sequelae.
- Clinically manifested by elevated peak airway pressures, decreased cardiac output, oliguria, septic complications from gut bacterial translocation and elevated intracranial pressures.

- Typically occurs when intra-abdominal pressures >25 mmHg.
- Bladder pressure is the standard method for measuring intra-abdominal pressure.

Management of the open abdomen

In the immediate postoperative period or immediately after decompressive laparotomy, coverage of the exposed intra-abdominal contents must be achieved (see Temporary abdominal closure below). In the later postoperative period, if it is impossible to close the wound then there are the following options:

1 Coverage of intestinal contents by approximating the skin edges. The ventral hernia is accepted and a planned repair at 6–18 months performed.
2 Allowing the exposed intestinal surface to form a bed of granulation tissue followed by split thickness skin grafting. A follow-up procedure for removal of the skin graft and repair of the hernia with abdominal wall component separation will be necessary.
3 Placement of vicryl (or other absorbable) mesh to the fascial edges, covering the exposed intestinal contents. A bed of granulation tissue is allowed to form followed by split thickness skin grafting. Hernia repair as above will be necessary.
4 Closure of the wound over time by secondary intention. Some patients may opt not to have further surgery and will accept the long-term issues of an incisional hernia.

'There is little point in achieving a technically excellent wound closure if the patient dies of the sequelae' Anon (2006).

Temporary abdominal closure

The open abdomen requires coverage of the exposed intra-abdominal contents and in the immediate postoperative period there must be adequate control of effluent. If fascial closure is not possible or inadvisable then there are many different ways to achieve this:

Skin closure

The skin may be closed over unapproximated fascia. This is the best option if possible, but it is important to avoid precipitating ACS by an overtight closure.

Occlusive dressings

Bogotá bag

First developed in Bogotá, Columbia in 1984, the Bogotá bag involves covering exposed bowel with a sterile silastic sheet (traditionally an opened out 3 L urological irrigation bag), which is then sutured to the surrounding skin (Figure 1.3). The most commonly used material in our centre are empty bags of 0.9% saline, divided at three edges and cut to shape.

'Vacpack' dressing/Opsite sandwich

Surgeons can construct a vacuum dressing that can be applied directly on to bowel (Figure 1.4):

- *Step 1.* Select a sterile towel of comparable size to the wound you wish to cover.
- *Step 2.* Wrap the towel in a sterile adhesive dressing, e.g. Ioban™.

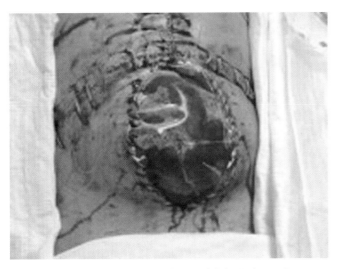

Figure 1.3 Bogotá bag *in situ*. *Partial* closure of abdominal wound at a second look laparotomy for severe liver trauma The subcostal incision had been closed while a Bogotá bag was used for the midline wound until a further attempt was made to close the wound at a third laparotomy.

- *Step 3*. Place the non-adhesive towel dressing in the wound, tucking the edges under the fascial edge. Jackson-Pratt (suction) drains are placed either side of the dressing at the fascial edge.
- *Step 4*. Cover the entire wound with a second large sterile adhesive sheet. Ensure that the drains are wrapped within a mesentery of the adhesive sheet to provide a good seal.
- *Step 5*. Finally, attach the proximal end of the drain to a suction source. This shrinks the dressing and wound overall and collects effluent.

KCI Vac dressing

Vacuum Assisted Closure device (V.A.C.® Therapy Kinetic Concepts Inc.™, San Antonio, Texas) is a non-adhesive proprietary dressing with a patented black sponge suction that acts to collect effluent fluid, shrink the wound and promote granulation tissue by inducing a uniform suction throughout the wound surface (Figure 1.5).

A piece of foam sponge with an open-cell structure is placed on to the abdominal wound and fashioned into shape. The entire area is then covered with a transparent adhesive membrane, which is

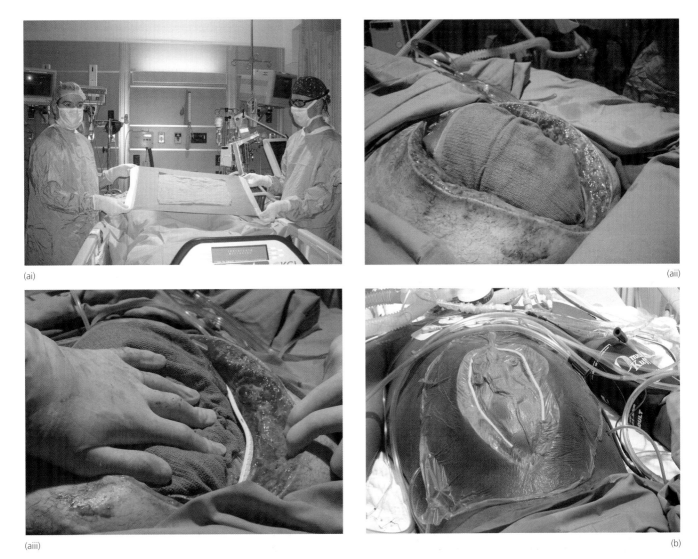

(ai)

(aii)

(aiii)

(b)

Figure 1.4 (a, i–iii) Constructing an Opsite sandwich. (b) An Opsite sandwich in place.

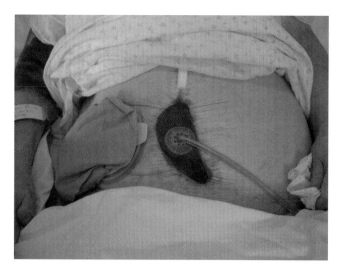

Figure 1.5 VAC dressing *in situ*.

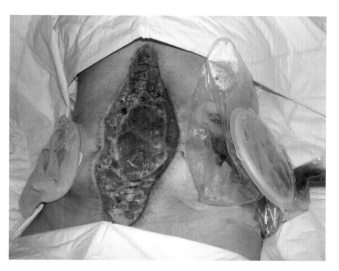

Figure 1.6 Complex abdomen.

firmly secured to the healthy skin around the wound margin. The adhesive membrane is perforated and a drain with lateral perforations is positioned on top of it and connected to a vacuum source. Fluid is drawn from the wound through the foam into a reservoir for subsequent disposal.

The plastic membrane prevents the ingress of air and allows a partial vacuum to form within the wound, reducing its volume and facilitating the removal of fluid. The foam ensures that the entire surface area of the wound is uniformly exposed to this negative pressure effect, prevents occlusion of the perforations in the drain by contact with the base or edges of the wound and eliminates the theoretical possibility of localized areas of high pressure and resultant tissue necrosis.

Tip

Stomas are best initially avoided with open abdomens. If a stoma is sited at the same time as performing a laparostomy with vacuum-assisted dressing, the stoma should be positioned in an extra-lateral position to allow adequate seal for the dressing. The adhesive membrane covering the abdomen should be placed on first, a hole is then cut out for the stoma and the stoma bag placed on top of this.

The complex abdomen

Management of the patient with a complex abdomen (Figure 1.6) following an intra-abdominal 'catastrophe', trauma or abdominal sepsis requires the full attention and close cooperation of the multi-disciplinary team. It is imperative that while in hospital a *named consultant* takes overall responsibility for directing care, surgical intervention and referral for opinions. A clear schematic drawing in the notes of the procedure(s) performed is vital for the rest of the team to provide information on lines, tubes, drains, stomas and options for feeding (Figure 1.7).

It is through attention to detail at all levels, and the coordination of surgery, imaging and radiological intervention (when indicated) and perseverance that the best results will be obtained.

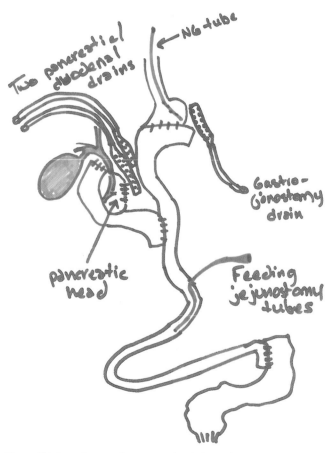

Figure 1.7 Operation note from a complex abdominal trauma. The drawing provides other surgeons and the team caring for the patient with clear information to help them manage the complexity of his postoperative care.

The complex abdomen patient often requires the coordination of therapies over a protracted time for some or all of the following:
- Critical care (surgical airways, intravenous lines, ventilation);
- Wound infection;

- Open abdomen;
- Multiple abdominal drains;
- Multiple operations;
- Repeat imaging;
- Interventional radiology (drainage of collections);
- Management of abdominal fistulae;
- Stoma care; and
- Nutrition (enteral and parenteral).

These patients often have long hospital stays and we have found it valuable to produce a summary of events and interventions every 50 days of hospital stay.

Further reading

Braslow B, Brooks AJ, Schwab CW. Damage control. In: Mahoney PF, Ryan JM, Brooks AJ, Schwab CW, eds. *Ballistic Trauma: A Practical Guide*. Springer-Verlag, Frankfurt, 2005: 180–208.

Schecter WP, Ivatury RR, Rotondo MF, Hirshberg A. Open abdomen after trauma and abdominal sepsis: a strategy for management. *Journal of the American College of Surgeons* 2006; **203**: 390–396.

World Society of Abdominal Compartment Syndrome. www.wsacs.org

CHAPTER 2

Surgical Airways

Andrew Taylor

OVERVIEW

- A surgical airway is a temporary or permanent opening through skin into the trachea
- Emergency cricothyroidotomy is a life-saving technique which all personnel who have contact with emergency or trauma patients should be familiar
- Minitracheostomy is an aid to clear secretions
- Tracheostomy is performed on critically ill patients requiring long-term respiratory support
- Care of patients with a tracheostomy involves many members of the health care team

Introduction

A surgical airway refers to the formation of a temporary or permanent opening through the skin into the tracheal lumen. This may be an emergency procedure to gain control of the airway (e.g. use of a cricothyroidotomy in severe facial trauma with airway obstruction) or an elective procedure (e.g. tracheostomy in the presence of severe head injury, anticipating a long requirement for ventilation and respiratory care).

- **Cricothyroidotomy is insertion of a tube or catheter through the cricothyroid membrane**
- **Tracheotomy is the creation of an opening in the trachea**
- **Tracheostomy is the formation of an opening between the trachea and the skin**

Cricothyroidotomy

All personnel who have initial contact with trauma and emergency patients should be skilled in cricothyroidotomy. Cricothyroidotomy is often a last resort procedure when other means of establishing an airway, such as endotracheal intubation, have failed, although in some military settings it may be used as the definitive airway of choice. It is a life-saving technique and involves making a puncture or incision through the cricothyroid membrane to allow oxygenation.

The reasons why establishing an airway may prove difficult include:
- Facial injury from severe trauma;
- Blood or vomit in the airway;
- Airway swelling from oedema or haematoma; and
- Obstruction due to foreign body or tumour

Synonymous terms with cricothyroidotomy include coniotomy or cricothyrotomy

Needle cricothyroidotomy

A large bore cannula (12–14 G) is inserted through the cricothyroid membrane into the trachea. This is then connected to either a low or high pressure oxygen supply. Needle cricothyroidotomy provides only temporary oxygenation (up to 30 minutes) but not ventilation because of the small internal diameter of the cannula lumen; in addition, the cannulae are prone to kinking. A needle cricothyroidotomy should be replaced with a definitive surgical airway as soon as possible (Figure 2.1).

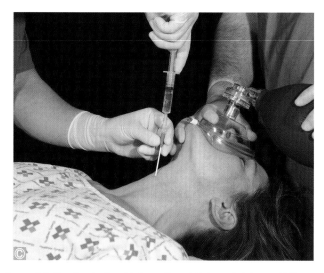

Figure 2.1 Needle cricothyroidotomy. From J Nolan, ed. *Advanced Life Support*, 5th edn. The Resuscitation Council (UK), London, 2006. © Mike Scott and Resuscitation Council (UK).

ABC of Tubes, Drains, Lines and Frames. Edited by A. Brooks, P. Mahoney and B. Rowlands. © 2008 Blackwell Publishing, ISBN: 978-1-4051-6014-8.

Surgical cricothyroidotomy

An endotracheal or tracheostomy tube is inserted through a transverse incision which is made through the cricothyroid membrane, using a scalpel blade. To minimize bleeding, it is recommended that a horizontal incision is made over the lower half of the cricothyroid membrane thus avoiding the cricothyoid artery. The advantage of a surgical cricothyroidotomy is that a small cuffed endotracheal tube (size 6 or 7) can be passed through the hole. This protects the airway and allows the patient to be effectively ventilated.

> Tracheostomy tubes should not be inserted through cricothyroidotomy incisions

Emergency cricothyroidotomy kits

These kits contain more rigid and wider bore cannulae specifically designed for cricothyroid puncture. They come pre-packaged with all the required components to enable the procedure to be performed quickly and efficiently. Most kits also incorporate a 15 mm connector, which allows the device to connect immediately to a standard breathing circuit. The Portex Emergency Cricothyroidotomy Kit (Figure 2.2) comprises a cuffed 6 mm tube and has been used extensively in the field by both ambulance crews and the military.

The complications of cricothyroidotomy include:
- Bleeding;
- Subcutaneous emphysema;
- Barotrauma/pneumothorax;

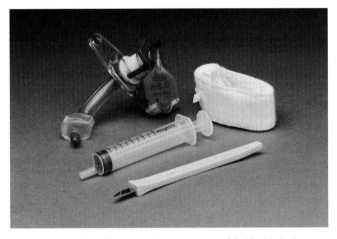

Figure 2.2 Cricothyroidotomy set. Image courtesy of Smiths Medical International Ltd.

- Oesophageal perforation; and
- Creation of a 'false passage' in the soft tissues of the neck.

Minitracheostomy

A minitracheostomy is a 4 mm internal diameter non-cuffed tube which is inserted through the cricothyroid membrane. Minitracheostomies are aids to clear secretions and are not licensed or intended for use as emergency cricothyroidotomy airways. Commercially available minitracheostomy kits are available, e.g. Minitrach II minitracheostomy (Smiths Medical International Ltd; Figure 2.3).

Tracheostomy

A tracheostomy is a transcutaneous opening in the trachea below the level of the cricoid cartilage. The tracheotomy should be made between the second and fourth tracheal ring to prevent complications of cannulation. Tracheostomy is performed routinely on intensive care units (ICU) for patients in whom long-term intubation is anticipated (Box 2.1).

The most common indications to perform tracheostomy are:
- To allow ventilation and facilitate weaning;
- To bypass an upper airway obstruction;
- To provide airway protection from aspiration; and
- To provide airway access during surgery.

The optimal timing to perform a tracheostomy remains controversial. It is usually considered if the duration of intubation is anticipated to be longer than 10–14 days. Complications of prolonged oral intubation include infection (sinusitis, ventilator-associated pneumonia), vocal cord damage, tracheal stenosis and tracheomalacia.

Percutaneous vs. surgical tracheostomy

Tracheostomies for patients on ICU were traditionally performed by a surgeon in theatre. In recent years, this has been superseded by

---

Box 2.1 **Benefits of tracheostomy**

- Increases patient comfort
- Facilitates weaning
- Allows reduction in sedation
- Facilitates clearance of tracheal secretions
- Reduces laryngeal and glottic trauma
- Facilitates speech
- Allows oral nutrition

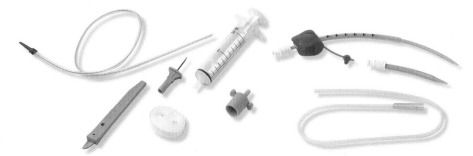

Figure 2.3 Minitracheostomy. Image courtesy of Smiths Medical International Ltd.

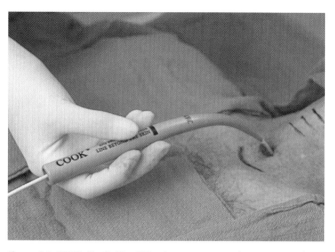

Figure 2.4 COOK Ciaglia Blue Rhino Percutaneous Tracheostomy Introducer Set. Image courtesy of Cook Incorporated, Bloomington, IN.

Box 2.3 **Types of tracheostomy**

- Cuffed/uncuffed
- Extra long/adjustable flange
- Non-fenestrated/fenestrated
- Armoured tubes
- Silver tubes (e.g. Negus)

a percutaneous technique. Percutaneous dilational tracheostomy (PDT) is procedure that can be performed at the bedside, without requiring the assembly of a surgical team and transfer to theatre.

The advantages of PDT are:
- There is minimal bleeding;
- There is a reduced risk of infection of the stoma;
- There is a better cosmetic result; and
- It can be performed almost immediately.

There are several methods of performing PDT, the most common of which was described by Ciaglia and colleagues in 1985. In the *Ciaglia* technique, the trachea is punctured by a needle, through which a guidewire is introduced. While this may be performed blindly, direct visualization of the needle and wire placement using a bronchoscope reduces the serious complications of the technique, such as posterior tracheal wall damage and para-tracheal placement. Once correctly positioned, multiple dilators of increasing diameter are then passed along the guidewire, generating a tissue track that is sufficiently wide to accommodate the tracheostomy tube. Figure 2.4 shows the 'Blue Rhino', which uses a single tapered dilator, instead of the sequential dilators described by Ciaglia. The dilator has a special hydrophilic coating, which once wet becomes slippery, easing the insertion of the dilator through the tissues.

In the Griggs technique, a pair of special dilating forceps is used to 'spread' the tissues, having been similarly advanced into the trachea over a guidewire. Despite being a rapid 'one-step' dilation, this technique is thought to be associated with a higher incidence of tracheal injury, and is less popular.

The surgical technique should be chosen in preference to the percutaneous technique where there are anatomical challenges, such as:
- Previous neck surgery;
- Cervical spine fracture;
- Obesity or short 'bull' neck; or
- Blood vessels overlying intended puncture site.

Tracheostomy tubes

The tracheostomy tube is *arc*-shaped (referred to as the *Jackson curve*) to allow the correct angle of entry into the tracheal lumen. Tracheostomy tubes are available in a variety of types, lengths and diameters (Box 2.3). They are also made of a number of different materials to suit each patient, including polyvinylchloride, silicone, silver and rubber (silastic).

Components of the tracheostomy tube

1 *Outer cannula.* This is the main body of the tracheostomy. The size of the tube usually refers to the inner diameter; 7–9 mm is satisfactory for most adults.
2 *Inner cannula.* This is a removable tube that fits within the outer cannula. The inner cannula is vital to prevent obstruction of the tube by mucus as it can be removed and/or replaced. It is recommended that it should be cleaned every 4–6 hours with warm running water and a brush. All patients on a general ward should ideally have an inner cannula.
3 *Cuff.* This is a balloon at the distal part of the tube and provides a seal between the tube and tracheal wall. The cuff can be inflated (to protect the lungs from aspiration and allow positive pressure ventilation) or deflated to allow speech.
4 *Pilot balloon.* This is an external balloon connected to the internal cuff by an inflation line. It gives an indication of whether the internal balloon is inflated.
5 *Flange.* The flange prevents the tube slipping into the trachea. It also provides an area to secure the tube to the neck with tapes, ties or sutures.

6 *15 mm connector.* This allows attachment of the tracheostomy to all adult standard breathing circuits.

7 *Introducer/obturator.* This is a rounded tipped shaft that is placed inside the outer cannula to reduce trauma during tube insertion. It is removed once the tracheostomy tube is inserted (Figure 2.5).

Cuffed tubes

Cuffed tracheostomy tubes are used for patients who require positive pressure ventilation or who are at risk of aspiration. The pressure exerted by the cuff can impair perfusion to the tracheal mucosa leading to necrosis and eventually stenosis. The pressure exerted by the cuff can be reduced by using 'high volume, low pressure' cuffs whereby the large volume distributes the pressure more widely (Figure 2.6). Cuff pressure should be limited to 15–25 cm H_2O, which can be checked with a manometer.

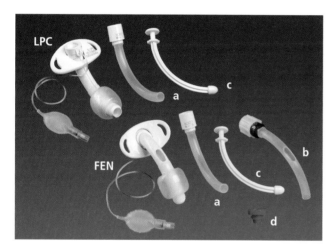

Figure 2.5 Tyco tracheostomy. LPC, cuffed tracheostomy cannula; FEN, fenestrated cuffed tracheostomy cannula; a, inner cannula; b, fenestrated inner cannula; c, obturator to facilitate insertion; d, decannulation plug. © 2006 Tyco Healthcare. All rights reserved.

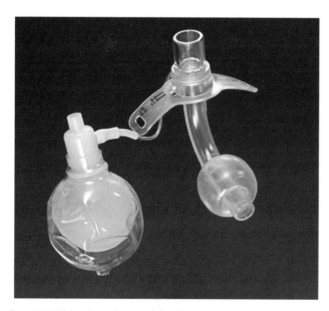

Figure 2.6 High volume, low pressure cuff. © 2006 Tyco Healthcare. All rights reserved.

Uncuffed tubes

Uncuffed tubes are used for patients who no longer need positive pressure ventilation and are no longer at risk of aspiration. An uncuffed tube allows voice production and swallowing. They do not have a pilot balloon (Figure 2.7).

Fenestrated tubes

Fenestrated tubes have single or multiple holes. The advantage of the fenestration is that it enables air flow to the larynx to allow the patient to speak. They are contraindicated in patients requiring ventilation because of air leakage through the hole.

Extra long tracheostomy tubes

Standard length tubes (60–90 mm) may not be suitable for patients with an increased skin to tracheal distance. Adjustable flange tubes are longer in length (up to 130 mm); the length can be varied by adjusting the position of the flange (Figure 2.8). Adjustable flange

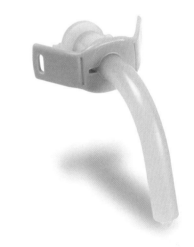

Figure 2.7 Uncuffed tube. Image courtesy of Smiths Medical International Ltd.

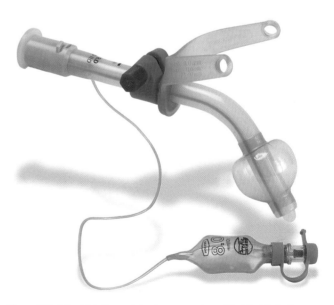

Figure 2.8 Adjustable flange tube. Image courtesy of Smiths Medical International Ltd.

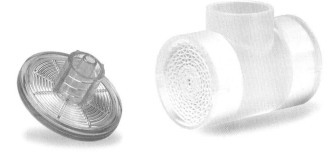

Figure 2.9 Heat and Moisture Exchangers. Image courtesy of Smiths Medical International Ltd.

tubes are not available with inner cannula and are therefore prone to occlusion.

Care of the patient with a tracheostomy

Humidification
Inspired air is normally warmed and moistened by the upper airways. This humidification is essential for normal respiratory function; air that is cold and dry damages the respiratory mucosa, impairs mucociliary clearance and the removal of secretions. All patients with a tracheostomy should receive humidified gases as the upper airway is bypassed. Methods to provide humidification include heat and moisture exchangers (HME, 'Artificial Nose' or 'Swedish Nose'; Figure 2.9), hot and cold water humidifiers and tracheal bibs.

Suctioning
Suctioning is essential to prevent the accumulation of secretions, which can block the tracheostomy tube, resulting in potentially fatal consequences. Suctioning stimulates the cough reflex; the frequency of suctioning depends on the amount and viscosity of secretions. Suctioning is associated with a number of serious complications, including hypoxia and cardiac arrhythmias. To minimize these, the patient should be pre-oxygenated and a maximum of three passes should be allowed each time. The entire procedure must never take more than 15 seconds. Suction pressures should be limited to 13.5–20 kPa to prevent damage to the tracheal wall.

> **The formula for choosing the right size catheter is:**
>
> **(size of tube [internal diameter] – 2) × 2**
>
> **e.g. 8 mm internal diameter (8 – 2) × 2 = 12 ∴ select a size 12 catheter**

Wound care
Meticulous care of the newly formed stoma site is essential to allow healing of the wound. The stoma site should be assessed daily; a healthy stoma appears red and moist with a healed edge. As the stoma site is in constant contact with secretions, it is at continual risk of maceration. Regularly removing these secretions is vital to prevent skin breakdown and infection. Specialized hydrophilic

foam dressings, designed to absorb moisture away from the skin, are available to keep the wound dry.

Communication
The presence of a tracheostomy tube impairs the ability to speak and communicate. Initial means of communication will almost always be non-verbal; for example, using mouthing, lip reading and writing. Utilizing the knowledge and skills of the speech and language therapists, who can give advice on the best means of communication, is essential. Voice production is achieved by directing airflow past the tracheostomy tube into the larynx. Techniques to enable voice production include:
- Cuff deflation;
- Using a fenestrated tracheostomy tube;
- Downsizing the tracheostomy tube;
- Intermittent tube occlusion;
- Speaking valves (e.g. Passy-Muir valve); and
- Talking tracheostomy tube (e.g. Vocalaid).

> **The cuff should always be deflated when a speaking valve is attached**

Speaking valve
These are one-way valves that are placed on the distal end of the tracheostomy. When the patient exhales, the valve shuts and air is redirected around the tracheostomy tube through the vocal cords. This will allow phonation, e.g. Orator speaking valve (Smith Medical International Ltd), Passy-Muir speaking valve (Kapitex; Figure 2.10).

Swallowing
Patients with tracheostomy tubes may have impaired swallow as a result of both mechanical and physiological effects of the tube on the swallowing mechanism. It is recommended that before oral nutrition is allowed the patient undergoes a swallowing assessment by the speech and language therapist. As a general rule, patients with inflated cuffs are kept 'nil by mouth'.

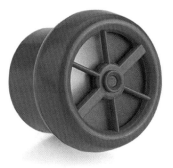

Figure 2.10 Passy-Muir speaking valve. © Copyright Kapitex Healthcare 2005.

Tube changes

The frequency of tube changes depends on the individual patient and amount of secretions being produced. Changing a tracheostomy tube carries significant risk. An anaesthetist or competent practitioner should always perform the first tracheostomy tube change. In all cases, it is important to note the outer diameter of the tube, especially if exchanging for different type or manufactured tubes.

> The first tube change should not be performed within 7 days to allow the stoma to establish

Decannulation

Decannulation is the removal of a tracheostomy tube. Before it is contemplated, it is important to ensure that the patient can maintain spontaneous breathing (for at least 24 hours), has successfully tolerated cuff deflation, can cough effectively and protect their airway, and is free from excessive pulmonary secretions. Following decannulation the patient should be monitored for 48 hours.

Long-term tracheostomy care

The successful discharge of a patient into the community who requires a long-term tracheostomy requires a collaborative interdisciplinary approach. The discharge process should provide support not only for the patient, but also many members of the community health care team, who may have limited experience of tracheostomy care. The aim is to return the patient to normal life, with as much independence as possible.

Further reading

Delaney A, Bagshaw SM, Nalos M. Percutaneous dilatational tracheostomy versus surgical tracheostomy in critically ill patients: a systematic review and meta-analysis. *Critical Care* 2006; **10**: R55 [abstract].

Durbin CG Jr. Techniques for performing tracheostomy. *Respiratory Care* 2005; **50**: 488–496 [abstract].

Homewood J, de Beer JMA. Tracheostomy care. *British Journal of Hospital Medicine* 2005; **66**: M72–M73.

Russell C, Matta B (eds) *Tracheostomy: A Multi-Professional Handbook.* Greenwich Medical Media, London/San Francisco, 2004.

St. George's Healthcare NHS Trust. *Guidelines for the Care of Patients with Tracheostomy Tubes.* Portex Limited, August 2000.

CHAPTER 3

The Chest

Ben Davies

OVERVIEW

- Cardiothoracic operations are common and the timely recognition of postoperative complications by non-specialist physicians is important
- Thoracic trauma is common
- The majority of significant thoracic trauma can be adequately managed by chest drainage
- Chest drain insertion is a vital diagnostic and therapeutic procedure and should be familiar to all involved in acute medicine and surgery
- If in doubt, ask a senior member of your team or consider contacting a thoracic surgical unit for advice
- Optimize postoperative recovery by ensuring adequate analgesia, early physiotherapy and dietitian referral

Introduction

The chest relies on the integrity of its wall and tissues to protect underlying structures and contribute to the physiology of breathing. Disruption of this integrity and function from pain, trauma or surgery may result in hypoxia.

Chest drains are used to drain free air and fluid from the chest cavity, help lung re-inflation and move the patient back towards a more normal physiology. Significant morbidity can be caused by inappropriate or incorrect chest drain placement, a procedure often delegated to junior members of the team. All practitioners involved in the management of the acutely unwell patient should be competent with this procedure.

Common chest incisions, wounds and aftercare

Table 3.1 lists thoracic incisions.

Complications

1 Wound-specific:
  - Superficial infection.
  - Sternal wire infection.

ABC of Tubes, Drains, Lines and Frames. Edited by A. Brooks, P. Mahoney and B. Rowlands. © 2008 Blackwell Publishing, ISBN: 978-1-4051-6014-8.

  - Suspected deeper infection (mediastinitis) and sternal dehisence.
  - Ipsilateral shoulder stiffness following thoracotomy. Encourage gentle shoulder movement.
  - Wound seroma. More common after muscle-sparing approaches due to skin flap development.
2 Rib fractures.
3 Neurological:
  - Intercostal nerve injury:
    Major cause of chronic post-thoracotomy pain; and
    Chronic pain >1 year uncommon (5% of patients).
  - Position-related brachial plexus injuries (uncommon). Paraesthesia in ulnar distribution can occur following median sternotomy. This usually settles spontaneously.
  - Superficial thoracic nerves:
    Long thoracic nerve – injury can lead to paralysis of serratus anterior 'winged scapula';
    Intercostobrachial nerve – at risk in vertical axillary thoracotomies and source of axillary paraesthesia.
4 Associated wounds and lines:
  - Leg wounds from saphenous vein harvest:
    Superficial infection (20–30%);
    Paraesthesia/neuralgia (25–30%);
    Seroma (uncommon).
  - Forearm wounds from radial artery harvest:
    Temporary sensory loss (variable);
    Permanent sensory loss (5–7%).
  - Feeding jejunostomy, e.g. following oesophagectomy or upper airways procedure.

Intercostal drains

Chest drains are a vital part of the management of chest trauma and elective cardiothoracic surgical procedures – few of these patients will escape without a chest drain. Their use in hospital is common but attention to detail is vital for successful management.

Indications for placement

- Air:
  'Simple' pneumothorax;
  Traumatic pneumothorax;
  Tension pneumothorax after initial needlethoracocentesis;

Table 3.1 Thoracic incisions.

Type	Access	Procedure
Anterior approaches		
Cervical		
Suprasternal	Superior/middle mediastinum	Mediastinoscopy
		Drainage of mediastinal/cervical root abscess
Transverse cervical	Trachea	Resection
	Thyroid/parathyroid	Thyroidectomy/parathyroidectomy
Thoracic		
Median sternotomy	Anterior mediastinum	Biopsy/resection
	Trachea, carina	Resection
	Both lungs	Uni/bilateral resections, lung volume reduction
	Heart	
Transverse sternotomy 'clamshell'	Anterior mediastinum	Resection
	Heart	Trauma
	Both lungs	Bilateral resections, lung volume reduction
		Lung transplantation
		Excision of extensive cervicothoracic tumours
Anterolateral thoracotomy	Lung	Limited resection/biopsy
	Heart (via pericardium)	Pericardial window/biopsy
Posterior approaches		
Posterolateral	Lung	Resection
	Oesophagus	Resection, myotomy, anti-reflux procedures
	Diaphragm	Hernia repair, plication
	Posterior mediastium	Tumour resection
	Trachea, carina	Resection
Lateral muscle sparing Thoracoabdominal	As per posterolateral	As per posterolateral
	Thoracoabdominal aorta	Aortic replacement
	Oesophagus, stomach	Resection and reconstruction

Persistent or recurrent pneumothorax after simple aspiration; Large spontaneous pneumothorax in patients >50 years.
- Fluid:
Haemothorax;
Pleural effusion;
Infected fluid (parapneumonic effusion or empyema);
Chylothorax.
- Others:
Rib fractures and positive-pressure ventilation;
Fractures often associated with underlying lung injury at risk of developing pneumothoraces;
Traumatic arrest (bilateral) – in case the arrest is due to tension pneumothorax.

Relative contraindications
- Bleeding diathesis;
- Anticoagulation therapy.

Aims of chest drainage
- Drain air and/or fluid from the pleural cavity;
- Re-expand the lung and obliterate residual spaces;
- Restore negative intrathoracic pressure.

Selection of chest drainage device
- Intercostal drain:
Infants and young children   8–12 French

Table 3.2 Chest radiography findings and their significance.

Finding	Action/implication
Pneumothorax	Chest drain or aspiration
Haemo/pneumothorax	Chest drain
Pneumomediastinum	Aerodigestive injury
	Potential for later mediastinitis
Widened upper mediastinal contour	Cardiac or vascular injury

Children and young adults   16–20 French
Adults   Air   24–28 French
            Fluid/blood 28–40 French
                  (28–36 French most commonly used)
- Seldinger-type drain.
- Redivac drains.
- Pneumodart.

How to insert a chest drain
- Where possible obtain verbal consent and pre-medicate with an opiate, benzodiazepine or ketamine.
- Check local policy for prophylactic antibiotics – consider in trauma case.

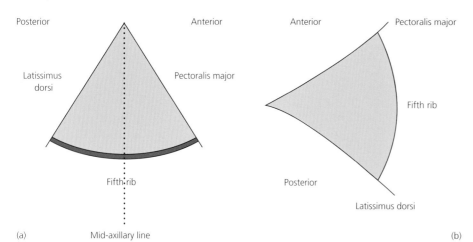

(a)   Mid-axillary line

(b)

Figure 3.1 (a,b) Triangle of safety. (b) Supine position.

- Locate triangle of safety (Figure 3.1).
  Landmarks:
  Anterior border of latissimus dorsi;
  Lateral border of pectoralis major;
  Horizontal line superior to level of nipple/fifth rib.
- Position patient to maximize access for yourself and in a position that they will comfortably be able to hold for a number of minutes.
- Glove and gown. Using aseptic technique, prep and drape the axilla and anterolateral chest wall widely.
- Aim for a site between the anterior and mid-axillary lines above the nipple/fifth intercostal space to avoid long thoracic nerve and breaching the abdomen, respectively. This approach only involves the intercostal muscles, allows mobilization and is preferred to alternative approaches that tether muscles, hamper chest wall movement and hence ventilation.
- If a thoracotomy scar is present, place drain superiorly to avoid the diaphragm which may be adherent to previous incision.
- Local anaesthesia (max. 3 mg/kg plain lidocaine). Raise skin bleb then infiltrate deeper layers, including the periosteum on top of rib before progressing through pleura into pleural cavity. Analgesia will be improved by placing intercostals blocks at the level of the proposed incision and a space above and below.

Conventional chest tube

Start with a full thickness skin incision. Make it big enough to admit one of your fingers.

Place and secure an anchoring suture at one end of the wound and a vertical mattress suture at its mid-point in preparation for the drain's later removal. A linear incision should be closed in a linear fashion using a vertical mattress suture; there is no need to convert this to a painful, slow-healing and puckered wound by using a 'purse string'.

Aim to create a slightly oblique track into the chest with the pleural entry point 1–2 ribs higher than the skin incision to aid closure upon removal.

Use a Kelly clamp to create a path for the drain, opening the jaws in parallel to the rib, gently spreading soft tissue and muscle before breaching the pleura.

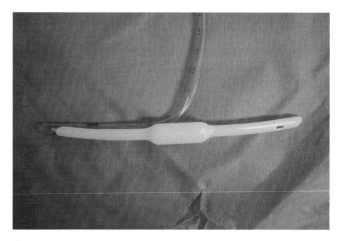

Figure 3.2 Disposable introducer.

Place a finger into the chest and sweep round, noting lung, adhesions or other structures that may be adherent to the chest wall so inadvertent damage can be avoided.

With the chest tube attached to either a Kelly clamp in parallel through a terminal drain hole or to a disposable introducer (*not* a trochar) introduce the drain into the pleural space, at which point the tube will start misting. Ensure all the holes in the chest tube are within the pleural cavity. Connect to chest drain system (Figures 3.2 and 3.3).

Percutaneous chest tube (Seldinger technique)

- Do not hesitate to make nick in skin to facilitate passage of the relatively blunt angled introducer needle.
- Orientate the needle.
- Aspirate as you go. Once you can pull back air or fluid, exchange the syringe for the guidewire and feed in gradually.
- Do not let go of the wire.
- Dilate over the wire.
- Run the drain over the wire.

This technique is considered by some to be less invasive, but prone to blockage and the requirement for regular flushing increases handling of the drains and increases the potential for intrapleural infection.

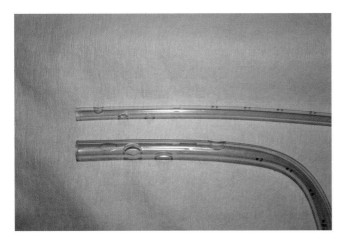

Figure 3.3 Drain holes.

Secure with pre-placed anchoring suture, apply sterile dressing over the area and confirm position with a chest radiograph. Avoid using thick tape such as Sleek™ which is difficult to remove quickly if you want to re-inspect in a hurry.

Top tips
- Avoid going too low (may injure diaphragm) or anterior (transfixing pectoralis minor or breast tissue).
- Do not underestimate movement of soft tissue when obese patient changes position; this can easily drag a carefully positioned drain out of the pleural space.
- Connect tube to a drainage system incorporating a one-way valve system and if possible, a calibrated collection chamber of which there are several types.

- Triangle of safety
- Blunt dissection
- No trocar. Finger first thing into the chest
- Consider prophylactic antibiotics, e.g. cefuroxime 750 mg

Drainage systems

Conventional underwater devices
Based on one, two or three bottles (Figures 3.4 and 3.5), in essence they are all similar, relying on a depth of water (usually 2 cm) to function as a one-way valve, allowing air and/or fluid out of the chest. Self-contained systems such as Atrium allow a predetermined maximum suction to be specified either by a mechanical valve (dry seal) or by adjusting the depth of water in a third chamber (akin to the third bottle).

Mobile device
The Heimlich valve was introduced in Vietnam in the 1960s. It is useful as one-way valve but is not able to contain fluid drainage. Contemporary portable devices cope with air and fluid, facilitating earlier mobilization and discharge from hospital, where appropriate. A flutter bag is often used in patients who have a small persistent air leak following lung resection (Figures 3.6–3.8).

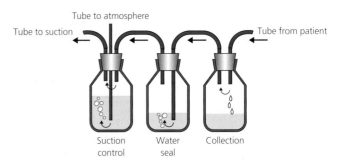

Figure 3.4 Three-bottle set-up.

Improvised device
In austere environments, temporary methods can be improvised, e.g. fixing a surgical glove with a fingertip cut off to the end of a chest drain.

Conventions and other information

Conventionally, chest tubes are directed apically for air and basally for fluid. In reality, provided there are no loculations, drain position in the chest probably does not actually matter as long as all of the holes are within the pleural cavity.

Following thoracic or upper gastrointestinal surgery, two or more drains may be in place. Convention dictates that the anterior drain is directed apically and emerges on the chest wall anterior to basally directed ones.

Small pneumothoraces, e.g. those detected on computed tomography (CT), may be managed conservatively in selected patients even if ventilated. If in doubt, discuss with your local trauma or thoracic surgical service for advice.

Further management – what to expect

Drain care
- Keep drainage device below the level of the chest at all times to prevent fluid siphoning back into the chest.
- Avoid dependent loops of tubing between the chest drain and the collection device.
- If the collection bottle foams, add a small amount (5–10 mL) of silicon-based defoamer to the collection chamber.
- Do not clamp a drain (unless testing for air leak or briefly while changing a bottle or connecting tubing).
- Swinging/oscillation of the water level with respiration indicates a patent drain in communication with the pleural cavity and reflects cyclical changes in intrapleural pressure.
- Persistent bubbling = air leak.
- Should an air leak occur, consider low pressure suction, typically −10 to −20 cm H_2O.

Drain removal
- Remove drain when:
  The lung is fully inflated;
  Bubbling or draining has stopped (<100 mL/24 hours), with minimal respiratory swing.

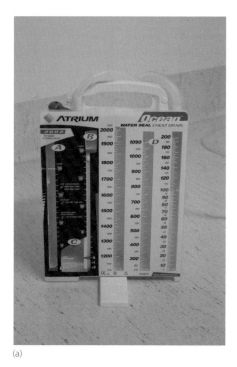

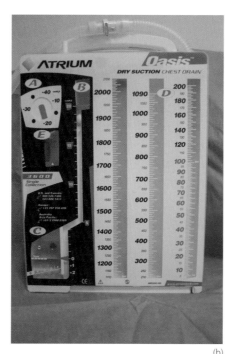

Figure 3.5 (a) Atrium water seal. (b) Atrium dry seal.

(a)

(b)

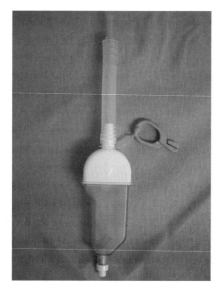

Figure 3.6 Mini collection.

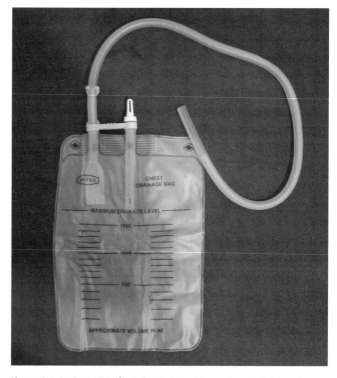

Figure 3.7 Drainage bag from the Portex military system with integral Heimlich valve.

- Remove at end-inspiration or during Valsalva manoeuvre, tie the pre-placed suture and apply an occlusive dressing.
- Repeat a chest X-ray to document the lung position.
- Ensure the patient's pain is well managed to maintain chest excursion and hence lung expansion.

Complications

Tube-related

1 *Pain*: This is the most common complication. Chest tubes are often cited as the most traumatizing procedure by patients, and sufficient suitable analgesia should be used such as intercostal blocks, pleural blocks, epidurals, opiate analgesia and regular non-steroidal analgesics and paracetamol.

2 Damage to underlying thoracic or abdominal structures:
- Lung, e.g. air leak, lung collapse, bronchopulmonary fistula;
- Visceral and diaphragmatic injury;
- Great vessels;

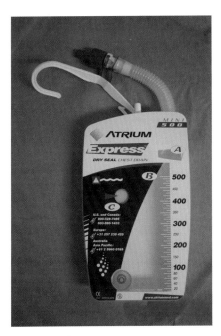

Figure 3.8 Portable dry seal.

- Thoracic duct;
- Neurological, e.g. long thoracic nerve injury, intercostal neuralgia.

3 *Displacement*: Usually occurs when the tube is not pushed in far enough initially. May be hampered by obesity and failing to anticipate movement of soft tissues to which the drain is anchored when sitting up or moving the patient's arm back down by their side. Manifests by development of surgical emphysema as drain holes bridge pleural space and soft tissues, allowing air to preferentially track into the tissues.

4 *Misplacement*: Extrathoracic placement can occur in obese patients, those with significant soft tissue oedema, e.g. (a third-spacing septic patient) or where the parietal pleura is abnormally thickened, e.g. in previous or active empyema.

5 *Infection*: Empyema occurs in 2–10% of patients who undergo chest drain insertion in the emergency department. In this situation, Gram-positive organisms are most common. Prophylactic antibiotics (e.g. third-generation cephalosporin) should be given for a minimum of 24 hours in such cases.

6 *Other*: Persistent air leak may occur in patients with a previous pneumothorax (on either side), a background of chronic lung disease, mechanical ventilation or acute respiratory distress syndrome (ARDS) either evolving or established (Tables 3.3 and 3.4).

Implications:
- Reduced effective tidal volume;
  Respiratory acidosis;
  V/Q mismatch;
  Inaccurate ventilator cycling information.
- Incomplete lung expansion.
- Dissipation of positive end-expiratory pressure (PEEP) throughout pleural cavity can further hamper lung re-expansion and worsen hypoxaemia.
- Risk of infection due to breach of respiratory tract.

Management of persistent air leak

Ensure chest drain(s) are sufficient to remove adequate volume of air. Consult with local thoracic specialist centre. Patients who are fit are best treated by video-assisted thoracoscopic surgery (VATS) with sealing of the air leak and pleurectomy to prevent recurrence.

Table 3.3 Persistent pneumothorax.

Air leak	No air leak
Airway injury	Extrathoracic chest drain
Chest drain displacement	Drain occluded
Large parenchymal injury	Lung re-expanded in area of drain holes
Pre-existing chronic lung disease, e.g. bullous emphysema	Airway obstruction
High airway pressures in ventilated patient	Lung collapse/consolidation
	Complete airway disruption with obstruction

Table 3.4 Types of air leak.

	Peripheral	Central
Alternative name	Parenchymal pleural fistula (PPF)	Bronchopleural fistula (BPF)
Source	Parenchymal	Breach at or proximal to segmental bronchi
Aetiology	Trauma Iatrogenic (chest drain) Barotrauma Purulent pulmonary infection	Traumatic major airway tear
Clinical features	Persistent bubbling in underwater drain Development of tension pneumothorax Worsening gas exchange manifests as respiratory distress	Persistent bubbling in underwater drain Respiratory collapse
Life-threatening compromise	Uncommon	Common
Treatment	Supportive	Repair airway tear

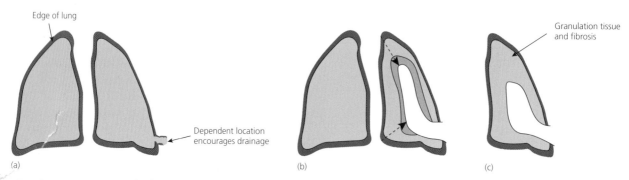

Figure 3.9 Thoracostomy. See text for further description.

This is effective in >95%, with most treatment failures evident within 30 days.

In patients who are unfit for surgery with persistent air leaks, the underwater seal may be changed to a flutter bag allowing them to be mobilized and discharged. Alternatively, sterile talc or autologous blood can be introduced via the indwelling chest drain as a form of pleurodesis to seal the leak.

Regional anaesthesia

Thoracic epidurals and intercostal or paravertebral catheters are commonly used peri- and postoperatively to provide balanced analgesia and optimize postoperative recovery, mobilization and pulmonary rehabilitation and mobilization of patients undergoing thoracotomy. They may also be used in multiple rib fractures or flail segments (for further details see Chapter 5).

Thoracostomy/'open thoracic window'

This is essentially a chronic stoma connecting the pleural space to the external environment and may be encountered in thoracic surgical practice or the district nursing environment. Provides a long-term solution to potentially life-threatening conditions. There are various eponymous names for it depending on the aetiology and surgical technique employed, e.g. Clagett window, Eloesser flap (Figure 3.9).

In essence, there exists free communication between the outside environment and the pleural cavity (Figure 3.9a). The mediastinum is fixed in position by fibrosis. The lining of the cavity itself tends to produce prolific granulation tissue, shrinking the cavity size (Figure 3.9b, c), a process that may be associated with relative reduction of the ipsilateral thoracic cage.

Indications

1 Infection:
 • *Empyema – especially if late presenting and unable to fully release/inflate lung at surgery;*
 • Suppurative lung disease; and
 • Following lung resection (post-pneumonectomy empyema).
2 Persistent space problem (following lung resection).

Considerations

• Pain/anaesthesia;
• Ongoing low-grade infection;
• Anticipate increased nutritional needs – refer to dietitian early, especially as such patients are already likely to be undernourished.

Further reading

Bojar R. *Manual of Perioperative Care in Adult Cardiac Surgery.* Blackwell Science, 2005.

Chikwe J, Beddow E, Glenville B. *Cardiothoracic Surgery (Oxford Surgery Handbooks).* Oxford University Press, 2006.

Deslauriers JJ, Mehran RJ. *Handbook of Perioperative Care in General Thoracic Surgery.* Mosby, 2005.

Karmy-Jones R, Nathens A, Stern E. *Thoracic Trauma and Critical Care.* Kluwer Academic Publishers, Netherlands, 2002.

Skinner D. *ABC of Major Trauma.* BMJ Books, London, 2002.

West JB. *Respiratory Physiology: The Essentials.* Lippincott-Wilkins, 2004.

CHAPTER 4

Lines

Adam Wolverson

OVERVIEW

- Lines are used for a wide variety of purposes:
  Administration of intravenous drugs
  Administration of intravenous nutrition
  Invasive cardiovascular monitoring
  Vascular access for specialized procedures
- Placement may be via needle over catheter or Seldinger techniques
- Central venous pressure (CVP) lines carry a higher risk of line site and catheter-related blood stream infection than peripheral lines related both to their location and prolonged use compared to peripheral intravenous (i.v.) lines.

Introduction

'Lines' refers to cannulae and catheters that are placed into the vascular system, most commonly inserted percutaneously into peripheral or central veins. Lines are used for a wide variety of purposes from short-term administration of intravenous drugs to the long-term administration of intravenous nutrition, for invasive cardiovascular monitoring and for vascular access for specialized procedures such as haemodialysis.

Peripheral intravenous lines

Peripheral intravenous (i.v.) lines are by far the most commonly used intravascular lines, and are widely used for vascular access in both hospital and pre-hospital practice (commonly referred to by the brand name Venflon – *BD Venflon*™) (Figure 4.1).

A peripheral i.v. line consists of a short plastic (polytetrafluoroethylene [PTFE]) cannula placed through the skin into a peripheral vein. Most cannulae have a connection port with a Luer lock fitting to allow connection to i.v. fluid administration sets and a one-way valve for the intermittent injection of i.v. drugs.

Occasionally, a needle itself may be inserted and secured into a vein for blood sampling or fluid administration (often referred

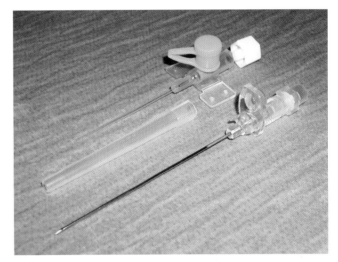

Figure 4.1 Photograph of basic intravenous (i.v.) cannula and compoment parts. Polytetrafluoroethylene (PTFE) cannula (i.v. portion). Hub with injection port and cover (for intermittent drug administration). Wings (for holding cannula during insertion/securing *in situ*). Luer lock port (for connection to i.v. fluid administration sets).

to as a 'butterfly'); these have the advantage of easier insertion but are not suitable for anything other than very short-term i.v. access.

For peripheral i.v. line insertion, a *cannula over needle technique* is most commonly used although a wire-guided Seldinger technique can be used for larger cannulae (Figure 4.2).

Size of i.v. lines

Intravenous cannulae come in a variety of sizes. The diameter of the cannula is the most important variable as this determines the flow rate of fluid via the cannula and is therefore used to define the size of the cannula. The size chosen will be dependent on both the intended use of the line and also the size of the patient's veins (Box 4.1).

Typically, cannulae are available from 22 G to 14 G; the lower the gauge the greater the diameter and the greater the maximum possible fluid flow rate. Smaller cannulae (22–20 G) are generally used for intermittent drug administration and larger cannulae (18–16 G) for i.v. fluid therapy, and very large cannulae

ABC of Tubes, Drains, Lines and Frames. Edited by A. Brooks, P. Mahoney and B. Rowlands. © 2008 Blackwell Publishing, ISBN: 978-1-4051-6014-8.

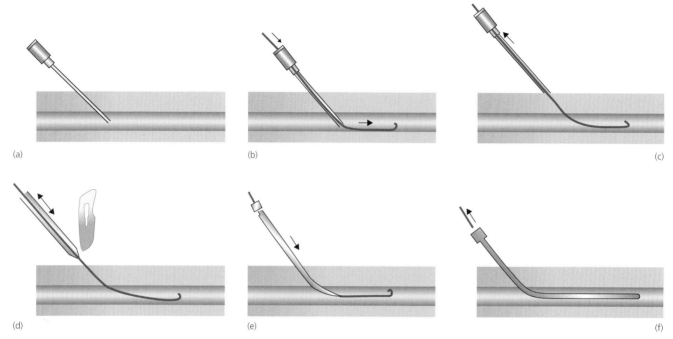

Figure 4.2 Seldinger catheter insertion. (a) Thin-walled needle introduced percutaneously into blood vessel. (b) Guidewire passed through needle and advanced into blood vessel. (c) Needle withdrawn leaving guidewire in place. (d) Skin puncture site enlarged with No. 11 scapel blade. (e) Catheter advanced over guidewire into blood vessel. (f) Guidewire withdrawn leaving catheter *in situ*.

Box 4.1 **Hagen–Poiseuille formula**

In any tube including i.v. lines the factors limiting flow are given by the Hagen–Poiseuille formula:

$Q = \pi Pr^4/8\eta l$

Flow = $\pi \times$ pressure gradient $\times$ radius^4/8 $\times$ viscosity of fluid $\times$ length of the tube

Therefore, for a given fluid and a given pressure gradient, flow is directly proportional to the fourth power of the radius of the cannula and inversely proportional to its length.

Typically, 22 G (0.9 mm) lines will have a maximal flow rate of around 40 mL/min, increasing to 270–300 mL/min in a 14 G (2.0 mm) line.

Box 4.2 **Measurement of catheter gauge**

Catheter gauges are conventionally measured either French (Fr/CH) or Gauge (G) systems.

French or Chaurie gauge
Used to express the external diameter of a catheter in 1/3 mm increments:

1 CH or Fr = 1/3 mm

Example: 6 CH or 6 Fr = 2 mm
 This unit is most commonly used for drain tubes, chest drains, etc, but is also used for some larger vascular access catheters. The larger the Fr/CH, the greater the diameter of the catheter.

British Standard Gauge or Standard Wire Gauge
Used to express the external diameter of a catheter, based on a system used to define the sizes of wires drawn from a standard sized metal rod. The numerical conversion into millimeters varies across the Gauge range, 8 G = 4 mm, 30 G = 0.3 mm. The larger the gauge, the smaller the diameter of the catheter.
NB: Neither system gives the internal diameter of the catheter which is the important variable in determining flow.

(14 G and larger) for rapid fluid administration during resuscitation. By convention in the UK, i.v. cannulae are colour coded based on their gauge.

A variety of cannula lengths are also available but typically narrower gauge cannulae are shorter in length (25 mm for a 22 G, increasing to 45 mm for a 14 G) (Box 4.2; Figure 4.3).

Sitting of peripheral i.v. lines

Peripheral cannulae can be sited in any accessible vein but most commonly veins in the back of the hand, forearm or antecubital fossa are used. Choice of site is determined primarily by the availability of a suitable vein for cannulation, but potential complications, patient comfort and ease of securing the line should also be considered.

Intra-arterial lines

Uses

Arterial lines are used for invasive blood pressure monitoring and to allow frequent blood sampling for arterial blood gas (ABG) analysis avoiding repeated arterial punctures. As an invasive technique with potential morbidity, their use is only justified when there is a

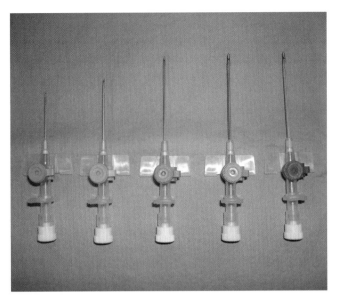

Figure 4.3 Intravenous (i.v.) cannulae sizes. By convention, i.v. cannula are colour coded based on their gauge: blue for 22 G, pink for 20 G, green for 18 G, grey for 16 G and orange–brown for 14 G. A variety of cannula lengths are also available but typically narrower gauge cannula are shorter in length (25 mm for a 22 G, increasing to 45 mm for a 14 G).

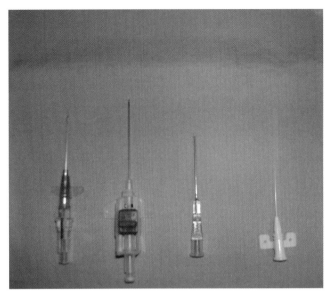

Figure 4.4 (from right to left) Arterial cannula; cannula over needle; Seldinger; Integrated guidewire (Arrow International™); Flow switch (BD Floswitch™).

need for continuous monitoring or frequent ABG analysis usually during anaesthesia or critical care admission. Use of arterial lines is limited to those areas of the hospital where staff are trained and experienced in their use and appropriate monitoring equipment is available.

Siting

The radial artery is most frequently used for arterial cannulation, if possible the non-dominant hand should be chosen. Dorsalis pedis arteries are also used particularly if repeated arterial cannulations are required in critical care patients. In patients who are peripherally shut down it may be necessary to site arterial lines in more proximal vessels, the brachial or femoral arteries, although these sites carry significantly increased risks of morbidity and should only be used in the short term and be replaced when placement in a more distal vessel is possible.

Type and size of arterial cannulae

The most commonly used are 20 or 22 G short (25–60 mm) arterial cannulae although cannulae up to 16 G and 15 cm in length are available. Both cannula over needle and Seldinger technique arterial cannulae are available as well as designs with an integrated guidewire to act as a guide for an over needle cannula (Arrow International™). Wire-guided arterial lines offer increased likelihood of successful arterial cannulation in patients with small or vasoconstricted vessels or in the presence of peripheral vascular disease (Figure 4.4).

Complications and care of arterial cannulae

The complications of arterial cannulation are significantly greater than those for peripheral venous cannulation. The risk of bleeding and haematoma formation at the insertion site are higher and infection is a significant risk. This means that meticulous asepsis at insertion and appropriate care of the line are vital. Arterial cannulae should be securely fixed *in situ* and be connected to a continuous low flow pressurized flush (normally flow is restricted to 3 mL/hour) to prevent backflow of blood and thrombus formation. The cannula should always be connected to continuous BP monitoring and alarms set should catheter disconnection occur.

Arterial cannulation has a potential for blood flow disturbance and tissue ischaemia from arterial occlusion or distal embolization of thrombus.

Central venous lines

Central venous pressure (CVP) lines are intravenous catheters place into the central veins (internal jugular, subclavian or femoral veins). They are used for a variety of purposes:
- To monitor central venous pressure and assess fluid resuscitation and cardiovascular status;
- To administer drugs that cannot be given via peripheral cannula (vasoactive drugs, chemotherapy, intravenous nutrition);
- To provide secure i.v. access for multiple drug infusions (during anaesthesia or in critically ill patients);
- To provide long-term access for i.v. therapy (long-term antibiotics, total parenteral nutrition); and
- For i.v. access when no peripheral veins are available for cannulation (burns patients, i.v. drug abusers).

Placement

CVP lines are most commonly placed percutaneously using a Seldinger technique. Traditionally, landmark techniques were used to identify the vein although now the use of bedside ultrasound is becoming routine. When the subclavian or internal jugular routes

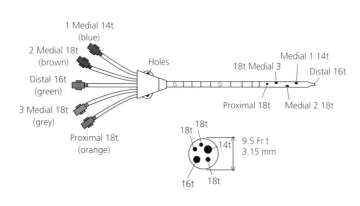

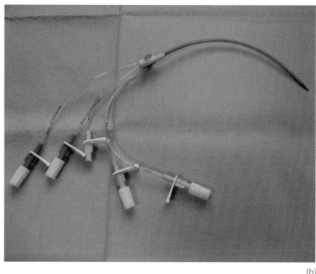

(a)   (b)

Figure 4.5 (a,b) Multi-lumen catheter sizes. Many central venous catheters are designed with multiple internal lumens to allow monitoring and multiple drug infusions simultaneously (usually 3, 4 or 5 lumens referred to as triple, quad or quin lumen lines, respectively). Each individual lumen has a separate connection hub on the external end of the catheter. On the intravascular portion each lumen ends in a separate opening or port. The distal port opens at the catheter tip, other ports then open onto the side of the catheter usually spaced at 1–2 cm intervals, the lumen that opens furthest from the catheter tip being referred to as the proximal lumen and lumens opening between distal are proximal as medial ports. For a typical 5 lumen CVP, the external catheter diameter will be 9.5 Fr (3.15 mm) containing a 16 G distal lumen, 1 1-G and 2 18-G medial lumens opening at 1, 2 and 3 cm from the tip and a proximal 18 G lumen opening 4 cm from the tip. With multiple lumen lines it is important to insert a sufficient length of catheter into the vein to ensure that the proximal lumen lies within the lumen of the vein to avoid extravasations of drugs or fluids given via the proximal lumen. Correct placement can be confirmed by aspiration of blood from all lumens, particularly the proximal lumen of the catheter.

are used, 10–15 cm of catheter is inserted so that the tip is ideally positioned in the superior vena cava just above the right atrium. When the femoral route is used the tip is place in the inferior vena cava usually requiring a catheter 25–30 cm in length.

CVP catheters are radio-opaque and post-insertion X-rays are obtained to ensure correct placement and detect potential complications.

CVP lines are available in a variety of lengths and gauges, and also as single or multiple lumen lines. Multiple lumen lines contain multiple separate lumens (2–5) within a single catheter and allow simultaneous monitoring and delivery of multiple drug infusions (Figure 4.5).

The site chosen for insertion of a CVP line depends on a balance of mechanical (e.g. bleeding, pneumothorax) and infective risks and the experience and training of the person inserting the line (Box 4.3).

CVP lines carry a higher risk of line site and catheter-related blood stream infection than peripheral lines, related both to their location and prolonged use compared to peripheral i.v. lines. Aseptic precautions should be employed for both insertion and ongoing care (Box 4.4; Figure 4.6).

Resuscitation lines

The primary requirements for i.v. lines for use in resuscitation after major trauma or haemorrhage is the ability to infuse high volumes of fluid or blood rapidly via a line that can be inserted both quickly and with low risk of complications.

Conventionally, two large bore (14 G) i.v. cannulae are recommended for fluid resuscitation, this will allow infusion of a total of approximately 500 mL/minute of fluid. Large cannulae are available for peripheral access, often referred to as emergency infusion devices (EID ™Arrow), typically 6 or 7 French (Fr) G and 4–5 cm in length, allowing very high fluid infusion rates. They can be rapidly inserted in a large peripheral vein using a Seldinger technique with a guidewire and dilator with a very low risk of complications.

Central venous access is not usually recommended for fluid resuscitation:

• Although multi-lumen central lines may be of large external diameter, the internal diameter of the individual lumens is usually no larger than that of conventional peripheral i.v. lines (18–14 G).

• CVPs line are significantly longer, often 25–30 cm in length, therefore flow rates via an equal gauge lumen will be significantly lower for a CVP line than a short (4–5 cm) peripheral line.

• Even in skilled hands CVP insertion takes significantly longer than siting peripheral i.v. access. The exception to this is in trauma centres with a high volume of trauma patients and where central placement of 8.5 Fr 'Sheaths' is the norm (see below).

• CVP lines are useful *after* initial resuscitation in order to assess the adequacy of resuscitation and monitor ongoing fluid requirements.

However, in some circumstances, such as in patients with severe limb injuries or who are peripherally vasoconstricted, it may not be possible to site peripheral i.v. access. In these circumstances either a surgical cut-down technique to access a peripheral vein or insertion of central venous access may be required.

Risks of CVP lines
- Infection (insertion site and catheter related blood stream infection [CRBSI])
- Pneumothorax
- Failed insertion/misplacement
- Haemorrhage (patients with coagulopathy/thrombolytic or anticoagulant drugs)
- Air emboli
- Pericardial tamponade/cardiac damage
- Cardiac dysrhythmia (direct catheter effect or cold/rapid fluid infusion)
- Venous thrombosis

Infection: subclavian has lowest relative risk, femoral lines highest
Pneumothorax: highest with subclavian, less with internal jugular, not with femoral
Failed insertion: subclavian is technically most difficult
Haemorrhage: clinically important bleeding most likely with subclavian (non-compressible insertion site haemothorax) and internal jugular

Relative risks of complications for CVP insertion sites

	Subclavian	Internal jugular	Femoral
Pneumothorax	+++	+	−
Haemorrhage	+++	++	+
Infection	+	++	+++
Pericardial tamponade	++	++	−
Dysrhythmia	++	++	−
Failed insertion	++	+	+
Air embolus	++	++	+
Venous thrombosis	+	+	++

Box 4.4 **Insertion and care of CVP lines**

On insertion
- *Asepsis*: prevention of contamination insertion site (hand hygiene, gloves, drapes and safe disposal of sharps)
- *Skin preparation*: alcoholic chlorhexidine gluconate allowed to dry for maximum effect
- *Catheter type*: single lumen unless multi-lumen line clinically indicated
- *Insertion site*: subclavian or internal jugular unless clinically contraindicated

Continuing care
- *Continuing clinical indication*: line still indicated and no indication for removal
- *Line insertion site*: regular observation for signs of infection, at least daily
- *Dressing*: intact, dry, adherent transparent dressing
- *Line access*: use aseptic technique and swab ports or hub with alcohol prior to accessing line for fluid or drug administration
- No routine line replacement unless clinically indicated

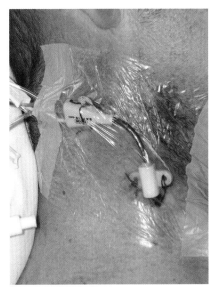

Figure 4.6 Adherent transparent dressing for CVP line.

Large gauge, single lumen, central venous catheters that will allow very rapid fluid infusion are available for this purpose, either specifically for resuscitation or as sheaths designed to allow the insertion of other intravascular devices such as pulmonary artery catheters (often refered to as Swan–Ganz sheaths). They have the advantages of being both large gauge (typically 8.5 Fr) and relatively short in length (10 cm), allowing very high fluid infusion rates.

Specialist i.v. lines

A variety of more specialized i.v. lines are available for specific purposes. These include:
- Lines allowing vascular access for haemodialysis and other forms of extracorporeal circulation;
- Tunnelled lines specifically designed for long-term central venous access for parenteral nutrition or chemotherapy;
- Vascular access sheaths designed to allow placement of transvenous pacing wires, angiography catheters and pulmonary artery catheters.

Haemodialysis lines

A number of therapies require passage of large volumes of blood via an extracorporeal circulation. Most commonly this is done for renal replacement therapies in renal failure (haemodialysis [HD] and continuous venovenous haemofiltration [CVVH]), but also for molecular absorbent recirculating system (MARS) in liver failure, extracorporeal membrane oxygenation (ECMO) in acute respiratory failure and for plasmaphoresis and plasma exchange.

Lines designed to provide access for these therapies allow high blood flows and usually consist of a dual lumen catheter placed in a central vein, with one lumen used to take blood out of the vein (conventionally labelled as the red 'arterial' lumen) to the extracorporeal circuit and the second lumen to return the blood to the patient (conventionally labelled as the blue 'venous' lumen).

These lines are typically 12 Fr in external diameter, 16–20 cm in length and contain 2 × 12 G lumen allowing blood flows of up to 340 mL/minute at the pressures used in extracorporeal circuits (up to 200 mmHg).

They are inserted in the same way as conventional CVP lines and can be placed at any site used for CVP access. Tunnelled and cuffed versions of the lines are also available for more secure long-term use, although for long-term haemodialysis the surgical formation of an arteriovenous shunt allowing intermittent access is usually preferred.

Long-term i.v. access lines

A number of therapies require long-term i.v. access, typically total parenteral nutrition (TPN), chemotherapy and occasionally long-term antibiotic therapy. These require venous access that is secure, carries a low risk of infective complications and allows the infusion of large volumes of fluid (1–3 L/day for TPN) into a large central vein. These lines are made of silicon and designed to be tunnelled subcutaneously from the site of insertion to a distant skin entry site (on the anterior chest wall) to reduce the infection risk.

To improve the security and further reduce infection risk, catheters are available with a Dacron cuff (Hickman lines) that sits subcutaneously near the skin entry site (Figure 4.7).

Totally implantable vascular access devices

As a further development of long-term tunnelled vascular catheters, totally implantable vascular access devices (TIVADs) have been developed to allow safe and effective long-term vascular access. These devices are similar to tunnelled central lines, but rather than having an access port that lies externally with the catheter passing through a skin entry site, TIVADs end with a titanium access chamber that is implanted beneath the skin and access to the catheter is gained by passing specially designed needles or cannulae through the skin and into the access chamber via a self-sealing membrane.

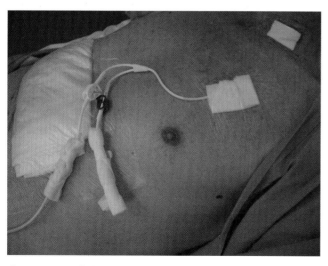

Figure 4.7 Tunnelled line.

Pulmonary artery catheters

A pulmonary artery catheter (Swan–Ganz) is a diagnostic instrument that allows advanced monitoring of the cardiovascular system by direct measurement of pressures in the right atrium, right ventricle, pulmonary artery and, indirectly, the filling pressure ('wedge' pressure) of the left atrium. It also allows measurement of other caridovascular parameters.

Pulmonary artery catheters have a number of indications and may be useful to differentiate cardiogenic shock, septic shock and hypovolaemia, in the management of complicated myocardial infarction, in the assessment and diagnosis of respiratory distress and pulmonary hypertension, in the management of vasoactive drugs and inotropes and fluid management in the critically ill.

The pulmonary artery catheter is introduced through an introducer sheath placed in a large central vein. From this entry site it is passed, with the aid of fluoroscopy or by observing the pressure trace recorded from the catheter tip, through the right atrium, right ventricle and subsequently into the pulmonary artery. Placement is facilitated by a small (2 mL) inflatable balloon at the catheter tip which carries the catheter into the pulmonary artery with the flow of blood through the heart. The balloon, when inflated, also causes the catheter to 'wedge' in a small pulmonary blood vessel. When 'wedged' the catheter then provides a measurement of the 'filling pressure' of the left ventricle of the heart.

Use of pulmonary artery catheters is not without significant risks, in addition to the usual risks of passing a large catheter in a central vein. Complications of its insertion have included arrhythmias, damaged heart valves and 'wedging' of the catheter can cause pulmonary artery rupture or distal infarction (Figure 4.8).

Care of lines and line infection

As with any indwelling device, all i.v. lines carry a significant risk of both local and systemic infection and correct care of i.v. lines both during placement and use is important, both to reduce the risk of infection and prevent the need for frequent re-siting (Box 4.5).

The risk of infection varies with:
- *Type of line*: CVP lines greater risk than peripheral venous and arterial lines;
- *Site of insertion*: greater risk with femoral lines than internal jugular and subclavian lines;
- *Duration of insertion*: risk of infection increases the longer a line is *in situ*;
- Number of *disconnections/reconnections* of infusions that are made.

Bacteraemia rates of peripheral lines have been estimated to be up to 3.7 per 1000 patients with a peripheral i.v. line or 0.2 per 1000 line days. Serious infections are more common with CVP lines and up to 6000 significant central venous catheter-related blood stream infections occur per year in England. For peripheral lines, available evidence supports re-siting lines after 72 hours; for CVP lines, however, available evidence *does not* support routine re-siting of lines in the absence of clinically suspected infection.

Redness, swelling and tenderness at an insertion site or along the line track, the presence of frank pus at the insertion site or positive blood cultures obtained from a line are all indicative of line infection.

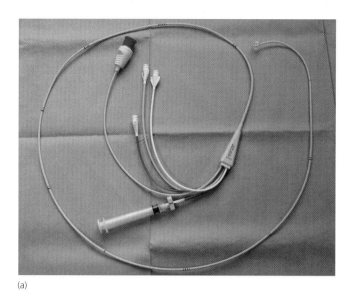

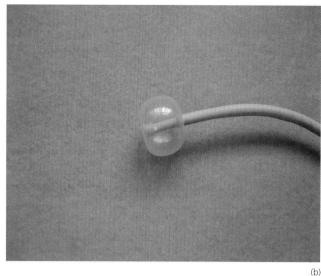

(a)

(b)

Figure 4.8 (a) Pulmonary capillary wedge pressure (PCWP) catheter. (b) Inflated balloon tip.

Box 4.5 **Insertion and care of i.v. lines**

On insertion
- *Asepsis*: prevention of contamination insertion site (hand hygiene, gloves, drapes and safe disposal of sharps)
- *Skin preparation*: 70% alcohol or alcoholic chlorhexidine allowed to dry for maximum effect
- *Dressing*: a sterile semi-permeable transparent dressing to allow observation of insertion site
- *Documentation*: date of insertion recorded in notes

Continuing care
- *Continuing clinical indication*: line still indicated and no indication for removal
- *Line insertion site*: regular observation for signs of infection, at least daily
- *Dressing*: intact, dry, adherent transparent dressing
- *Line access*: use aseptic technique and swab ports or hub with alcohol prior to accessing line for fluid or drug administration
- *Administration set replacement*: immediately after blood, blood products or lipid feed, after 72 hours for all other fluids

However, intravascular lines may be infected in the absence of any of these localizing signs and present only as systemic sepsis.

In cases of sepsis of unknown origin, blood cultures should be taken from all intravascular lines that have been *in situ* for 48 hours or more and consideration given to removing any line that may be the source of infection. In clinically suspected or proven line infection the line should be removed and if necessary replaced at another site. Replacement at the same site by rewiring an *in situ* line is not adequate and should not be undertaken as the line may be infected.

Removal of CVP lines

Removal of CVP lines carries a risk of bleeding from the insertion site and possible air embolus. CVP lines should be removed with the patient in a position where the insertion site is below the level of the heart (i.e. head down for internal jugular and subclavian lines) to reduce the risk of air embolus. Firm pressure with sterile gauze should be applied to the site until bleeding has ceased and the site then covered with a sterile dry dressing.

CHAPTER 5

Pain

Trudy Towell and Jonathan Mole

OVERVIEW

- Pain perception is a complex process that is affected by a variety of inputs around the body
- Repeated assessment of pain is fundamental for delivering good analgesia
- Multimodal analgesia improves pain relief
- Early and effective pain relief may reduce morbidity and mortality
- Understanding the mechanism and risks of particular interventions will improve their safety and effectiveness

Introduction

Our understanding of pain has undergone a number of changes in recent years. The traditional description of a 'hard-wired' system of a peripheral painful stimulus transmitted uninterrupted to the brain does not reflect the complexity and plasticity of neural transmission, nor does it account for the 'second stage' when the brain creatively transforms impulse patterns into perceptual qualities, emotions and meanings.

Broadly, two approaches to pain have evolved. The 'bottom-up' approach traces the painful stimulus activating a pain receptor (nociceptor), which sends a signal up the primary afferent neurone to synapse in the spinal cord and then up to the brain. It then looks at how this pathway is influenced (Figure 5.1).

The 'top-down' approach starts with people's descriptions of their pain as the brain does more than detect and analyse sensory inputs; it creates perceptual experience even in the absence of external inputs so that we do not need a physical injury to feel pain.

Delivering effective analgesia for the surgical patient requires individual assessment and planning, an understanding of the pathophysiology of acute pain, the use of multimodal therapy and a team approach that involves a substantial educational and organizational effort.

Assessment

History

Previous pain experiences, fear, anxiety, depression, coping styles, cultural background, social supports and meaning attached to the pain all interact to produce the pain described by patients. Explanations and reassurance are therefore very important.

Assessment

Assessment of the patient's pain and recording its response to treatment is fundamental to good pain control (Figure 5.2). The best methods involve self-reporting rather than observer assessment. Simple verbal rating scales (pain score of 1–10, mild/moderate/severe) are reasonably reliable as long as frequent assessments and recording are undertaken. Assessment of common side effects such as sedation, hypotension and nausea are also important. For procedural pain, especially if it is to be repeated, assessments are needed before, during and after the procedure to optimize techniques. Planning of analgesic strategies takes place alongside assessment.

Postoperative analgesia

The effective treatment of acute pain is a fundamental component of quality patient care. Failing to relieve severe pain can be harmful in many ways, physiologically and psychologically (Box 5.1). Conversely, effective treatment of postoperative pain (sometimes including pre-emptive analgesia) may reduce the incidence of postoperative morbidity. Better treatment of postoperative pain may also lead to decreased levels of chronic pain. This requires a team approach and a focus wider than analgesic drugs alone.

Principles of acute pain management:
- Involvement of the individual in assessment and control of pain;
- Early treatment, because established pain is more difficult to treat;
- Multimodal analgesia;
- Adequate education of carers and patient;
- Local guidelines but tailored to the individual; and
- Follow-up assessment and charting of pain and possible side effects.

Multimodal analgesia

The combination of different classes of drugs; non-steroidal anti-inflammatory drugs (NSAIDs), paracetamol, local anaesthetics,

---

ABC of Tubes, Drains, Lines and Frames. Edited by A. Brooks, P. Mahoney and B. Rowlands. © 2008 Blackwell Publishing, ISBN: 978-1-4051-6014-8.

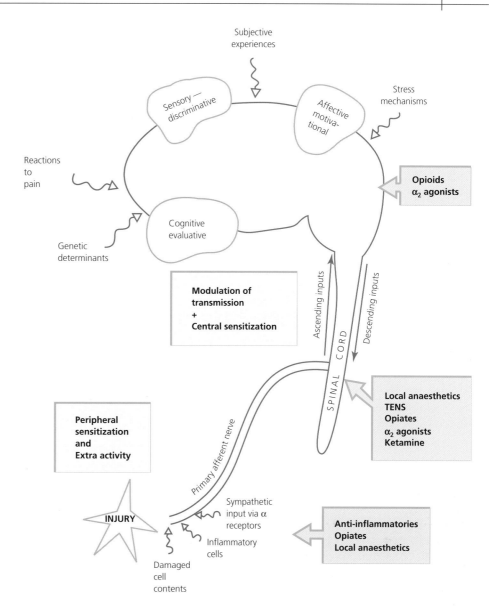

Figure 5.1 Pain sensation: pathways and intervention sites.

opioids and other non-opioid analgesics (e.g. clonidine, ketamine, gabapentin) improves pain relief and reduces the incidence and severity of the side effects of other drugs. This is the concept of 'balanced analgesia'. For example, the concurrent use of paracetamol significantly reduces the need for opiates. The World Health Organization (WHO) promotes the three-step analgesic ladder, which specifies treatment based on the intensity of pain. The oral route is preferred, but a variety of routes are available (e.g. subcutaneous, transdermal, rectal, intramuscular, intravenous, intrathecal, epidural and inhalational).

The remainder of this chapter deals with the practical mode of delivery of analgesia and the related lines and indwelling catheters that are associated with these techniques.

Intermittent subcutaneous opiate injection

The subcutaneous route has become popular in the management of acute pain, especially for opioids when the oral route is not suitable. A small cannula is inserted into the subcutaneous tissue and covered with a transparent dressing (usually in the upper arm, thigh or abdomen). The route and date of insertion should be clearly labelled (Figure 5.3):

- Subcutaneous is as effective as the intramuscular route and has a similar rate of absorption;
- Subcutaneous is less painful for the patient than intramuscular and reduces the risk of sharps injury;
- It is given over 1 minute;
- Can give hourly monitoring if appropriate;
- Change site if redness, swelling or persisting pain on injection;
- Unpredictable absorption if the patient is cold/shut down;
- May be as good as patient-controlled anaesthesia if done well (Figure 5.4).

Patient-controlled analgesia

A bolus of a fixed dose, commonly 1 mg morphine, is delivered intravenously by a pre-programmed secure pump when the patient activates it using a button (Box 5.2). A preset lockout period

Time (24 hour clock)								
Pain = X Sedation = 0	Ask patient to deep breathe, cough, move — score worst pain: moderate/severe pain requires action							
Severe	Unrousable							
Moderate	Sedated/rousable	O						
Mild	Drowsy	X						
None	Alert/awake							
Sleeping	**= Z** (rouse if resps <10)							
Nausea = **N**	Vomit = **V**	N						
Antiemetic given	**Y/N**	Y						
PCA bolus	Tries Good	✓						
PCA total volume infused								
Analgesia given	**Y/N**	N						
Bowels open	**Y/N**	Y						
Initials		AB						

Figure 5.2 Pain assessment chart. This is from the Queen's Medical Centre, Nottingham, and is used on the wards routinely. © Queen's Medical Centre, Nottingham University Hospitals Trust.

Box 5.1 Complications of traumatic/postoperative pain

Respiratory
Unrelieved upper abdominal pain leads to muscle splinting and:
• Hypoventilation, atelectasis (regional lung collapse), V/Q mismatch and hypoxaemia
• Poor clearance of secretions, lobular/lobar collapse and pneumonia
• Poor compliance with physiotherapy
Unrelieved lower abdominal and limb pain leads to immobility and:
• Hypostatic pneumonia

Cardiovascular
Severe acute pain causes sympathetic overactivity:
• ↑ Cardiac work and possibly ↓ myocardial oxygen supply and resulting ischaemia/infarction
• ↓ Peripheral circulation; with ↑ coagulability and immobility, leads to ↑ risk of thrombosis

Gastrointestinal and genitourinary
↑ Sympathetic activity leads to:
• ↓ Motility, possibly gastric stasis and paralytic ileus
• ↑ Urinary sphincter activity and role in urinary retention

General stress response
Acute pain contributes to this response especially in the early phases:
• Predominance of catabolic hormones
• Changes in coagulation and fibrinolysis
• Changes in water and electrolyte handling
• Increase in anxiety

(commonly 5 minutes) and the need for a conscious patient to activate the bolus are in-built safety features. When used in conjunction with an infusion (e.g. maintenance fluids), a non-refluxing valve should be used to prevent backflow and subsequent inadvertent opiate administration. Alternatively, a separate cannula can be used (Figure 5.5).

The patient accepts responsibility for the control of his/her own pain which in part explains the high patient satisfaction with this technique. Nursing or medical staff are not required to deliver analgesia and the patient can time bolus delivery to match changing needs, e.g. in anticipation of activity or a painful procedure. However, it is essentially a maintenance technique, and i.v. bolus doses may be required if opiate levels drop, e.g. after period of sleep. It is not appropriate if the patient is physically or cognitively unable to press the button in need.

Epidural analgesia

Insertion of the catheter is usually planned to be central to the incision/dermatomes to be blocked (e.g. T7–10 for upper abdominal surgery and L1–4 for hip/knee; Figure 5.6).

Advantages
In the appropriate patient, it can provide excellent analgesia postoperatively:
• May diminish a predominant part of the physiological response to surgical procedures, especially if there is complete alleviation of pain.
• Epidural analgesia reduces pulmonary complications, the duration of paralytic ileus after major abdominal surgery and thromboembolic complications after lower limb surgery.

Disadvantages
It is associated with a number of potentially very significant complications.
• Risk of epidural haematoma and epidural abscess with possible spinal cord damage (0.5–2 in 10,000 risk); the latter manifesting even after discharge. A high index of suspicion is needed followed by prompt investigation with magnetic resonance imaging (MRI).
• Puncture of the subarachnoid membrane with leakage of cerebrospinal fluid (CSF) may produce a severe, mostly self-limiting, headache of 24–48 hours duration (1 in 100–200 risk).
• Coagulopathy – *a contraindication* – will complicate catheter insertion and removal.
• Anticoagulant medications: a relative contraindication. Catheter removal and insertion checked against the time that anticoagulant drugs have been given
• Sepsis – catheter placement in the presence of sepsis may result in central nervous system (CNS) infection and/or epidural abscess.
• Hypotension – due to vasodilation.
• Respiratory depression – if the block is too high and interferes with respiratory muscles.
To minimize risk and maximize benefit, follow-up and monitoring is necessary by adequately trained staff with early detection of problems.

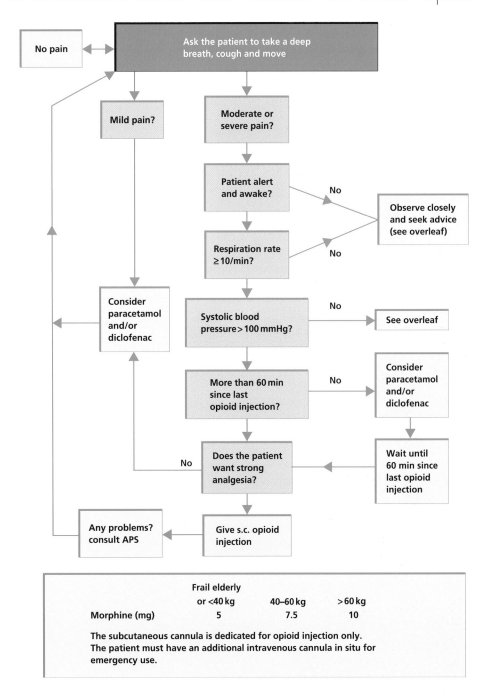

Figure 5.3 Algorithm for subcutaneous opiate administration. This is from Queen's Medical Centre pain department and is used in the Nottingham University Hospitals Trust. © Queen's Medical Centre, Nottingham University Hospitals Trust.

Within the figure:

- No pain
- Ask the patient to take a deep breath, cough and move
- Mild pain?
- Moderate or severe pain?
- Patient alert and awake? → No → Observe closely and seek advice (see overleaf)
- Respiration rate ≥10/min? → No
- Consider paracetamol and/or diclofenac
- Systolic blood pressure > 100 mmHg? → No → See overleaf
- More than 60 min since last opioid injection? → No → Consider paracetamol and/or diclofenac → Wait until 60 min since last opioid injection
- Does the patient want strong analgesia? → No
- Any problems? consult APS
- Give s.c. opioid injection

	Frail elderly or <40 kg	40–60 kg	>60 kg
Morphine (mg)	5	7.5	10

The subcutaneous cannula is dedicated for opioid injection only. The patient must have an additional intravenous cannula in situ for emergency use.

Action

- Infusion of local anaesthetic agent (LA) +/– opioid into epidural space via fine plastic catheter.
- LA blocks sensory nerves but also autonomic and motor nerves which can lead to hypotension and leg weakness.
- Opioids act directly on receptors in the spinal cord to provide analgesia without autonomic or motor block.
- Opioids can also produce respiratory depression by action on the respiratory centre via systemic absorption or upward diffusion in CSF.
- The combination of LA and opioid is synergistic, providing better analgesia on movement than either agent alone, but there is no particular combination that is clearly superior.

Considerations for securing catheter

(Figure 5.7)

- A bacterial filter is attached to the catheter for drug administration.
- Catheter is looped to prevent outward migration when catheter under tension.
- Some suture the loop, but this may encourage tracking of infection subcutaneously.
- Some tunnel catheter 5–10 cm. This may prevent dislodgement and probably delays tracking of infection when prolonged use.
- A transparent dressing allows daily inspection of insertion site. Look out for infection (erythema, pus, swelling), dislodgement (catheter markings of depth), leakage around and blood inside catheter (Table 5.1).

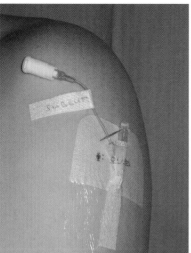

Figure 5.4 Subcutaneous cannula for opiate administration.

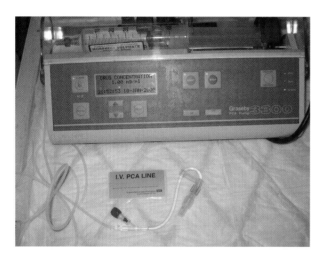

Figure 5.5 Anti-reflux and anti-syphon valves are present and the use is clearly labelled. The infusion pump is secure and pre-programmed.

Box 5.2 **Precautions for opiates**

Precautions for opiates:
- Need regular observations and assessment with protocol for dealing with problems
- Note that increasing sedation score is the earliest sign of respiratory depression. A low respiratory rate is a late and unreliable sign
- Need oxygen, naloxone and anti-emetics prescribed
- Extra care with patients with respiratory disease (including obstructive sleep apnoea) and allow for slow clearance in patients with renal impairment
- Ensure anti-syphon device on i.v. line if drip attached to same cannula for i.v. opiates
- Remember adjuvant analgesics for balanced analgesia and reducing opiate demand

Local anaesthetic agents

Traditionally used for short simple surgical procedures and interventions such as line and drain placement (Figure 5.8).

Wound infusor pumps

Recent interest has developed in the use of elastomer wound infusion pumps to prolong the LA effect. These supply a controlled continuous infiltration of the wound with a weak solution of LA for 24–72 hours postoperatively. These systems have been used in hip and knee replacement in order to reduce hospital length of stay through reduction in opiate analgesia used. They have also been used for amputation stumps and laparotomy wounds.

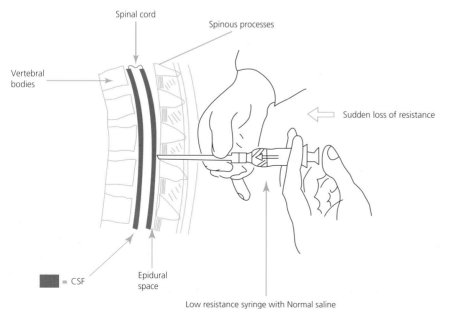

Spinal cord

Spinous processes

Vertebral bodies

Sudden loss of resistance

= CSF

Epidural space

Low resistance syringe with Normal saline

Figure 5.6 Epidural insertion. The resistance to injection from the ligamentum flavum is lost as the needle tip enters the epidural space.

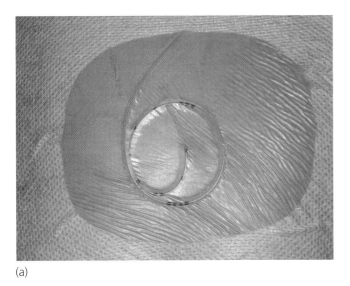

(a)

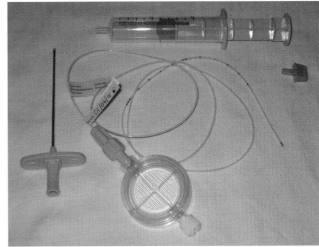

(b)

Figure 5.7 (a) Epidural catheter fixation. (b) A Portex epidural catheter kit.

Table 5.1 Troubleshooting for epidurals.

Problem	Possible cause (s)	Intervention
Hypotension	High block (>T4) Inadequate fluid replacement Ongoing blood loss	Lie patient flat, elevate legs, give oxygen Vasopressor, e.g. ephedrine 6 mg/4 min Fluid bolus (colloid/blood) if hypovolaemia Stop/reduce infusion if block >T4 (nipple line)
Inadequate analgesia	Catheter misplacement/migrated Missed segment Inadequate spread of block	Bolus from infusion and increase rate Bolus opioid (e.g. fentanyl 50 µg) Bolus LA, e.g. 0.25% bupivacaine 3–8 mL Re-site epidural Increase frequency observations for 30 min post intervention
Respiratory depression/oversedation	Sedation score increase is earliest sign, low resp rate is late and unreliable sign	Reduce infusion rate (sedation score 2, RR >8) Reduce rate, inform anaesthetist, consider naloxone (sedn score 2, RR <8) Naloxone 0.2 mg i.v., stop infusion, inform anaesthetist (sedn score 3)
Arm weakness/numbness	Epidural block too high	Stop infusion, measure BP
Persisting or increasing leg weakness	Epidural haematoma/abscess	Consider urgent MRI and neurosurgical review
Back/foot pain	Local bruising around site Epidural haematoma/abscess	Review MRI/neuro Sx as above
Fever and local spinal warmth/tenderness	Epidural abscess	MRI/neuro Sx as above
Severe itching	Opioids	May respond to naloxone 0.1 mg
Nausea and vomiting	Hypotension Opiate side effect	Check BP; see above Anti-emetics
Urinary retention	Autonomic block	Urinary catherization for retention, but not needed prophylactically unless indicated by surgery

LA, local anaesthetic agent; MRI, magnetic resonance imaging; RR, respiratory rate.

Nerve blocks/neural blockade

Blocking peripheral nerves with LAs provides analgesia for the whole area supplied by the nerve(s), not simply the area infiltrated. Femoral nerve blockade in the groin will numb a variable area down the anterior and lateral aspect of the thigh, as well as part of the hip and knee joint. Combinations of single nerve blocks, such as the 'ankle block', can extend the area anaesthetized. If the block is placed more proximally, before nerve bundles divide, as with brachial plexus blocks, then analgesia can be obtained over an even wider area. The duration of analgesia is longer than infiltration and

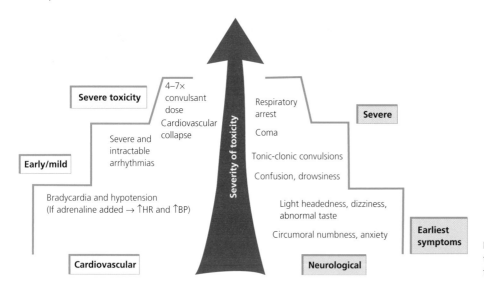

Figure 5.8 Symptoms of local anaesthetic toxicity. Note, with newer, racemic mixtures the pattern of symptoms may be different.

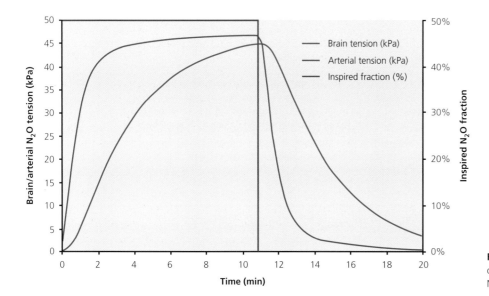

Figure 5.9 Entonox wash in curve. Courtesy of John Hardman. © Queen's Medical Centre, Nottingham University Hospitals Trust.

can provide excellent postoperative analgesia for up to 24 hours, in the appropriate patient, with a low risk of side effects. It can also be prolonged by the use of adjunct drugs and nerve sheath catheters.

Knowledge of anatomy is essential for choice of block and placement. Use of nerve stimulators helps locate nerves fairly accurately, but recent interest has focused on ultrasound visualization of the needle tip, in addition, which may allow more reliable blocks with smaller volumes of LA.

Safety aspects

- Pain or resistance on injection are warning signs of damaging intraneural injection. If possible, perform block on awake patients and inject at lower pressure with 20 mL syringe and with less traumatic 'block' needle.
- Avoid if coagulopathy or sepsis at injection site.

- Support affected limbs and inspect for adequate circulation; the painful symptoms of a developing compartment syndrome may be masked.
- Take care with initial mobilization in case weakness and impaired balance are present.
- Ongoing weakness/numbness, although it usually resolves, should be assessed and followed up.
- Establish oral analgesia before the block wears off.
- May mask painful symptoms of developing compartment syndrome.

- **Use of nerve stimulators helps locate nerves**
- **Ultrasound visualization of needle tip also used and may allow more reliable blocks with smaller volumes of local anaesthetic agents. Nerve sheath catheters and adjunct drugs can prolong the block**

Box 5.3 **Features of nitrous oxide**

Entonox/nitrous oxide (Figure 5.9)
- Analgesic and anaesthetic properties
- Long and safe track record outside theatre (including Queen Victoria)
- Commonly as 'Entonox' (50 : 50 mix of oxygen and nitrous oxide)
- Inhaled by activating a demand valve – a vital safety feature

Clinical features
- Short onset and offset
- Minimal respiratory and cardiovascular depression
- Effective analgesia and anxiolysis in adults and children, such as for labour pains, dental surgery, burns dressings, biopsy, venous cannulation
- Useful temporizing measure; awaiting epidural or while blocking nerves for traumatic injury
- Used alone or in combination with local anaesthetic agents and other analgesics

Box 5.4 **Troubleshooting for discharge pain**

- Check no shearing movement from poorly fixed drain
- Does the pain mean something (e.g. leakage round catheters/drains as sign of blockage or migration)?
- New, increased pain or changed in character needs assessment. Consider onset of neuropathic pain
- Septic symptoms (e.g. fever)
- Other symptoms (e.g. dyspnoea, new/deteriorating neurology, evidence of ischaemia)

Box 5.5 **Case history**

A 79-year-old woman was found 8 hours post laparotomy to be hypotensive and in pain, in particular around upper abdominal drainage sites. Her epidural infusion was stopped as a precaution and an on-call doctor was called to assess. Starting with assessment, her epidural sensory block level was found to be below the top of her wound and below the drain sites. The epidural had been working previously and there was no evidence of leakage around the insertion site. A low urine output and inadequate fluid replacement regime and clinical assessment pointed to hypovolaemia rather than a high block as the cause of hypotension, confirmed by a blood pressure improvement with an i.v. fluid bolus. After an epidural top-up bolus of local anaesthetic, her pain was assessed again and showed a marked improvement, with a now higher sensory block level. Regular paracetamol was prescribed in addition and an increase to the background rate of epidural infusion to maintain an adequate block.

Wherever possible, the oral route should be used: by the mouth, by the clock, by the ladder. The aim with postoperative pain relief is to go down the analgesic ladder, weaning off opiates with a baseline of paracetamol +/– NSAID (if not contraindicated). It is important to commence analgesia regularly prior to removing epidural intravenous patient-controlled analgesia, or before nerve blocks wear off.

If patients are to be discharged home with tubes, drains, lines or frames *in situ* it is important to provide verbal and, when available, written information to the patient and carers. Warning signs would include increasing analgesia requirements or new pain, signs of ischaemia and infection (Box 5.4).

Further reading

Allman K, Wilson I. Acute pain. In: *Oxford Handbook of Anaesthesia*, 2nd edn. Oxford University Press, 2006: 1025–1054.

Acute Pain Management: Scientific Evidence, 2nd edn. National Health and Medical Research Council (NHMRC) of Australia, 2005.

Grewal S, Hocking G, Wildsmith JAW. Epidural abscesses. *British Journal of Anaesthesia* 2006; **96**: 292–302.

Macintyre PE, Ready LB. *Acute Pain Management: A Practical Guide*, 2nd edn. W.B. Saunders, 2002.

Melzack R, Wall PD, eds. *Handbook of Pain Management*. Churchill Livingstone, 2003.

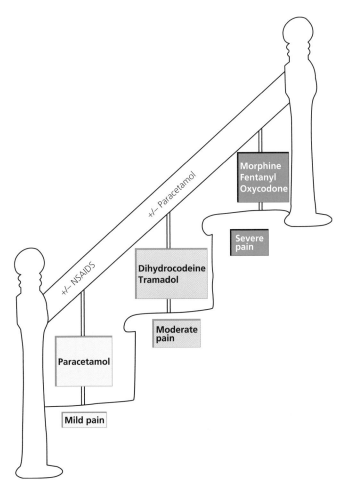

Figure 5.10 Modified analgesic ladder.

Step-down analgesia and discharge

The analgesic ladder recommended by WHO is a simple way of understanding pain management using analgesics (Figure 5.10).

CHAPTER 6

Feeding

Gabriel Rodrigues, Joy Field and Dileep Lobo

OVERVIEW

- If the gut is functional, enteral feeding is the method of choice
- Absolute indications for parenteral feeding include:
  - Intestinal failure
  - Short bowel syndrome
- Guidelines for enteral tube feeding are available
- Catheter-related sepsis occurs in 5–8 per 1000 patient days and is associated with morbidity, mortality and increased medical costs

Introduction

An inability to maintain an adequate oral nutrient intake either leads to malnutrition or puts the patient at risk of malnutrition. If the gut is functional, enteral feeding is the method of choice. Parenteral nutrition is indicated in patients with intestinal failure. In some patients, especially those with partial intestinal failure, enteral nutrition may be supplemented with parenteral nutrition to achieve adequate nutrient delivery. This chapter deals with indications for artificial nutritional support (Box 6.1), routes of delivery and care of feeding tubes and lines.

Enteral feeding tubes

Most enteral feeding tubes are made of polyurethane or silicone. Polyurethane is stronger than silicone and polyurethane tubes have thinner walls and thus a larger internal diameter, despite the same French gauge. The flexibility and decreased internal diameter of silicone tubes may lead to clogging or kinking of the tube. Tubes that are too flexible may be chilled before placement to increase stiffness (Figure 6.1).

Tube feeding

Enteral tube feeding can be accomplished via a nasogastric (NG) tube or by placing various tubes in the stomach or small intestine

Box 6.1 **Indications for artificial nutrition**

Enteral feeding
- Protein–energy malnutrition with inadequate oral nutrient intake for 5 days or more
- Less than 50% of required nutrient intake orally for 5–7 days
- Severe dysphagia
- Coma/stroke
- Low output enterocutaneous fistulae
- Cachexia
- Pancreatitis
- Severe orofacial trauma
- Burns
- Sepsis
- Liver failure
- Renal failure
- Preoperative nutrition
- Postoperative (e.g. oral cancers, oesophagus)
- Inflammatory bowel disease

Parenteral feeding
Absolute indications
- Intestinal failure
- Short bowel syndrome

Relative indications
- Complex enterocutaneous fistulae
- Moderate or severe malnutrition
- Acute pancreatitis
- Abdominal sepsis
- Prolonged ileus
- Major trauma and burns
- Severe inflammatory bowel disease

(Box 6.2). Some of the National Institute for Clinical Excellence (NICE) guidelines are summarized in Box 6.3.

Nasogastric tube

A nasogastric (NG) tube is inserted through a nostril, down the oesophagus into the stomach. It is suitable only for relatively short-term use as it is uncomfortable and tends to be removed by the patient. The placement of the tube should be checked frequently and the head end of the bed elevated to 30° during and after feeding to reduce the risk of aspiration.

ABC of Tubes, Drains, Lines and Frames. Edited by A. Brooks, P. Mahoney and B. Rowlands. © 2008 Blackwell Publishing, ISBN: 978-1-4051-6014-8.

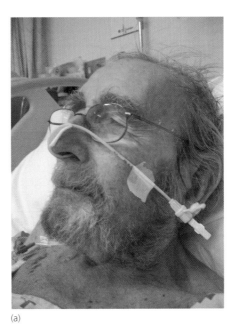

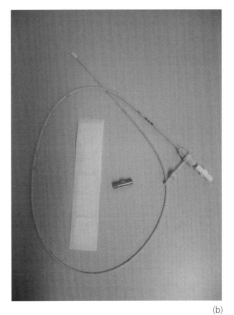

Figure 6.1 (a) Fine bore feeding tube *in situ*.
(b) Fine bore feeding tube kit.

(a)

(b)

Box 6.2 **Types of enteral feeding tubes**

• Nasogastric
• Nasojejunal
• Percutaneous endoscopic gastrostomy (PEG)
• Percutaneous endoscopic jejunostomy (PEJ)
• Surgical gastrostomy/jejunostomy

Box 6.3 **NICE guidelines for tube feeding**

• A functional and accessible gastrointestinal tract is a prerequisite
• Feeding should be stopped when oral intake is adequate
• Malnourished patients about to undergo major abdominal procedures should be considered for preoperative enteral tube feeding
• Nasogastric feeding is preferred unless there is gastric dysfunction or the stomach is inaccessible, in which case post-pyloric (duodenal or jejunal) feeding should be considered
• Gastrostomy feeding should be considered in people likely to need long-term (4 weeks or more) tube feeding
• In those with delayed gastric emptying who are not tolerating enteral tube feeding, a motility agent should be considered, unless there is a pharmacological cause or suspicion of gastrointestinal obstruction
• Consider post-pyloric enteral tube feeding and/or parenteral nutrition in prokinetic agent failure

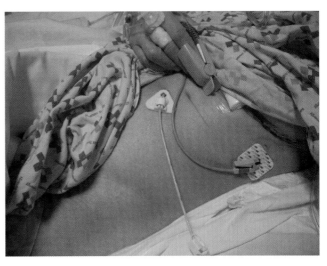

Figure 6.2 Percutaneous endoscopic gastrostomy (PEG) feeding tube.

into the stomach and are then propelled into the duodenum/ jejunum by peristalsis. However, most nasojejunal tubes are inserted under endoscopic or radiological guidance.

Gastric feeding tubes

Percutaneous endoscopic gastrostomy

Percutaneous endoscopic gastronomy (PEG) tubes come in a variety of sizes (9–24 Fr) and types (Figure 6.2). For younger patients there are also 'button' gastrostomies, which are aesthetically more acceptable. Another advantage to the 'button' type is that a restless patient, e.g. with cerebral irritation, is less likely to pull it out accidentally and cause displacement compared with the external tube present on a conventional PEG.

An uncorrected coagulopathy is a contraindication to placement of a PEG. Prophylactic antibiotics are usually given prior to this procedure. Post procedure, the patient remains nil by mouth and

Nasojejunal tube

Nasojejunal tube feeding is ideal for short-term access in patients in whom NG feeding is not feasible, e.g. where there is gastric outflow obstruction, in patients with pancreatitis and those at risk of aspiration from NG tube feeding. Some have two lumens, one for feeding into the jejunum and the other for aspiration of gastric contents. Some tubes, such as the Bengmark tube, can be inserted nil by PEG for 4 hours, after which the feed is commenced by flushing it with sterile water. Routine postoperative observations are recorded. Unless contraindicated (e.g. in spinal injury), the patient should be positioned with the head end elevated to 30–45° when feeding is in progress to prevent reflux and aspiration.

PEG removal

This can be carried out endoscopically or non-endoscopically. Once the internal balloon is deflated and collapses to a size that is small enough to allow its removal through the abdominal wall, gentle external traction will aid its removal. A fistulous tract may persist for a 2–3-week period which will eventually close down. If a PEG is removed accidentally, it is possible to insert a fresh tube or even a Foley catheter as an emergency measure through the tract until a PEG can be formally replaced and feeding can recommence.

Surgical gastrostomy

Gastrostomy tubes can also be placed during open or laparoscopic procedures. The most commonly performed is the 'Stamm gastrostomy' – a tube is passed through a small incision and into the stomach through the centre of the purse string sutures. They are suitable for long-term use, last about 6 months and can be replaced through the existing passage without an additional procedure.

Jejunostomy

A jejunostomy tube is similar to a gastric tube, has a finer bore and smaller diameter and can be introduced during open surgery or laparoscopically. Percutaneous endoscopic jejunostomy (PEJ) is an alternative to an open procedure if long-term post-pyloric feeding is required. The introduction of a feeding jejunostomy during major abdominal surgical procedures allows early postoperative enteral feeding and often saves patients from having to undergo intravenous feeding should complications arise postoperatively. Jejunostomy tubes can remain in place for a prolonged period, are effective and discreet and they are easily managed in hospital or in the patient's own home.

Care of the tubes

1 *Confirming the position*: The position of all tubes should be confirmed after placement (X-ray or aspiration of gastric contents). Guidelines from the National Patient Safety Agency (NPSA 2005) advocate aspiration of gastric contents before each feed and the use of pH graded indicator paper. A pH <5.5 is consistent with gastric placement.
2 *Fixing the tube*: The NG tube is usually fixed either to the nasal ridge or to the maxilla with a non-allergenic fixative tape and the tube is hooked over the ear. The gastrostomy and jejunostomy tubes have an inner radio-opaque fixation device (soft flange/balloon) that sits against the anterior abdominal wall. Externally they are fixed with a purse string silk suture. The idea is to prevent kinking and smooth delivery of the feeds and to prevent the tubes from being displaced. If the fixation suture loosens or cuts through, the tubes should be restitched immediately under local anaesthesia.

3 *Dressings*: Absorbable dressings should be applied around the exit site of the tube and need to be changed regularly, if soaked, to prevent skin excoriation/ulceration.
4 *Flushing*: This is essential before and after feeds. Blockage might require changing the tube which is a painful procedure. If blocked, fizzy liquid (e.g. soda water, lemonade or bicarbonate of soda) can be used to unblock the tube, or diluted pancreatic enzymes. Thin, firm and blunt wire stylets can also be used to clear the blockage.

Complications of feeding tubes and their management are summarized in Tables 6.1 and 6.2.

Methods of feeding

Tube feeds can be administered by bolus, continuous drip or a combination of the two. The best is a combination of oral and tube feeding.

Table 6.1 General complications of nasoenteral tubes.

Large bore tubes	Fine bore tubes
Nasopharyngeal discomfort and nasal bleed	Misplacement
Sinusitis and otitis media	Displacement
Necrosis/erosion of nasal cartilage	Blockage
Oesophagitis	Poor flow with viscous feeds
Oesophageal erosions/perforation	Difficult aspiration
Oesophageal stricture	Knotting
Rupture of oesophageal varices	Oesophageal perforation
Gastro-oesophageal reflux	
Gastric erosions/perforation/haemorrhage	
Duodenal perforation/haemorrhage	
Intussusception	
Pulmonary aspiration/pneumonia	
Lung collapse	
Tube misplacement	
Tube withdrawal	

Table 6.2 Percutaneous endoscopic gastrostomy (PEG): Complications and management.

Common PEG problems	Action
Stoma site infections	Swab site
Weeping and redness at insertion site	Course of antibiotics Adhere to local policies for care of site Usually settles with these measures
Tube blockage	Flush well before and after feeds and medicines If blocked, diluted pancreatic enzymes can be used or fizzy liquid, e.g. soda water or lemonade or bicarbonate soda
Over granulation	Silver nitrate carefully applied

Bolus feeding

This is delivered 4–8 times per day; each feeding lasting about 15–30 minutes. The advantages of bolus feedings over continuous drip feeding are that bolus feedings are more like a normal feeding pattern, more convenient and less expensive, if a pump is not needed. They also allow freedom of movement for the patient. However, the disadvantages are that reflux and aspiration may be more frequent than continuous drip feeding and in some cases they may cause bloating, cramps, nausea and diarrhoea. It may not be practical to bolus feed a patient when the volume of feed is large.

Continuous drip feeding

This may be delivered without interruption for an unlimited period of time each day. However, it is best to limit feeding to 18–20 hours or less. Feeding round the clock is not recommended as this limits mobility of the patient and may elevate insulin levels contributing to hypoglycaemia. Commonly, it is used for 8–10 hours during the night for volume-sensitive patients so that smaller bolus feedings or oral feeding may be used during the day. It is delivered by either gravity drip or infusion pump, the latter being better. The flow rate of gravity drip may be inconsistent and therefore needs to be checked frequently.

The advantage of continuous feeding over bolus feeding is that it may be tolerated better by children who are sensitive to volume, are at high risk for aspiration or have gastroesophageal reflux. Continuous feeding can be administered at night, so it will not interfere with daytime activities. It also increases energy efficiency, allowing more calories to be used for routine activities. When feeds are delivered continuously, stool output is reduced, a consideration for the patient with chronic diarrhoea. Continuous infusions of elemental formulae have been successful in managing patients with short bowel syndrome, intractable diarrhoea, necrotizing enterocolitis and Crohn's disease. The disadvantage of continuous feeding is that the patient is 'tied' to the feeding equipment during the infusion and it is more expensive because of the cost of the pump and additional feeding supplies that may be necessary.

The complications of enteral feeding and remedial measures are summarized in Table 6.3.

Parenteral feeding

Parenteral nutrition (PN) is used in gastrointestinal failure on a temporary or permanent basis and should only be used when it is impossible to meet nutritional needs via the oral or enteral route (Figure 6.3).

The required nutrients, electrolytes, trace elements, vitamins and water along with sources of energy and nitrogen are compounded under sterile conditions (laminar flow) in pharmacy into a large collapsible bag, usually 3 L in capacity. It is administered via an infusion pump either continuously over 24 hours or cyclically over 12–16 hours. Cyclical infusions can have physiological and psychological advantages. PN should be administered via a dedicated feeding line via a volumetric pump. Routes for access for parenteral feeding and some factors that determine the route for access are listed in Boxes 6.4 and 6.5.

Table 6.3 Complications of enteral feeding and their management.

Problem	Action
Diarrhoea	Exclude *Clostridium difficile* Usually due to antibiotics or other medications including laxatives Contaminated feeds, adhere to local policies/procedures, use sterile 'closed' feeding systems
Constipation	Review medications, i.e. opiates Give adequate fluid, hydration Treat in usual way with laxative
Vomiting/aspiration/inhalation	Position patient 30–45° unless contraindicated Give anti-emetic or prokinetic May need to reduce flow rate of feed If above fail may need consider NJ instead of NG feeding
Refeeding syndrome	Avoid overfeeding especially in very malnourished – 20 kcal/kg for first 24 hours and then slowly increase over 1/52 period Monitor biochemistry K, Ca, P, Mg Supplement K, Mg, PO_4 and thiamine Correct any imbalances Watch for signs of oedema

NG, nasogastric; NJ, nasojejunal.

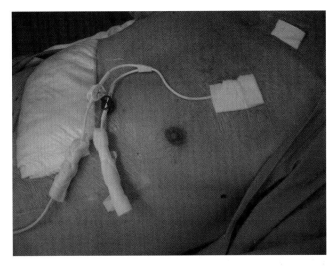

Figure 6.3 Hickman line ready for parenteral feeding.

Box 6.4 **Access for parenteral feeding**

- Peripheral parenteral nutrition (PPN)
- Peripheral inserted central catheters (PICC)
- Central venous catheter (CVC)
- Hickman/Borivac, cuffed or tunnelled lines

A variety of locations can serve as sites for catheter insertion including subclavian, internal jugular, femoral and cephalic veins. Due to the hyperosmolarity of parenteral solutions, the catheter tip must always be positioned into the superior vena cava (or inferior vena cava if a femoral line is inserted) so that the solutions

Table 6.4 Problems with access routes.

Access	Disadvantage
Internal jugular	Local hematoma Arterial injury Catheter-related sepsis higher than with subclavian route
Subclavian	Pneumotharax/haemothorax
Femoral	Very high risk of venous thrombosis and catheter-related sepsis
Peripheral veins	Thrombophlebitis Malposition Difficult insertion

Table 6.5 Some complications associated with parenteral feeding.

Insertion complications
Failure to cannulate
Pneumothorax
Air embolism
Arrhythmias
Haemothorax
Thoracic duct injury
Arterial puncture

Line-related complications
Infection (catheter-related sepsis)
Catheter damage/occlusion
Extravasation
Catheter-related thrombosis

Feeding-related complications
Metabolic (including refeeding syndrome and hyperglycaemia)
Cholestasis
Liver steatosis

are immediately diluted to tolerable concentrations. Solutions containing 10% or less dextrose (final concentration) plus amino acids (750–900 mOsm/L) can be infused into a peripheral vein (PPN). However, this is associated with a high risk of phlebitis and is therefore reserved for short-term therapy in individuals with robust veins. Simultaneous infusion of lipid emulsions will dilute the osmotic load and thereby improve tolerance to peripherally administered parenteral nutrition. PPN is useful for preserving somatic and visceral protein reserves in patients with limited tolerance of enteral nutrition support. Problems with parenteral access are listed in Table 6.4 and some complications associated with parenteral feeding are summarized in Table 6.5.

Management of catheter-related complications

Catheter-related sepsis
This occurs in 5–8 per 1000 patient days and is associated with morbidity, mortality and increased medical costs. It may present with a high swinging fever, a fever that subsides when the drip ends or pus at the catheter site.

To reduce the incidence:
- Use complete barrier precautions during insertion, skin preparation with chlorhexidine
- Never use prophylactic antibiotic ointment at catheter exit site
- PN lines should be reserved only for PN and handled by trained personnel

Management:
- Lock central venous line with sterile heparinized saline (HepSal)
- Start peripheral line, obtain blood cultures
- Examine for other sources of infection
- If cultures negative, restart infusion
- If cultures positive, remove line, send catheter tip for culture

Catheter occlusion
This can be recognized by the need to apply more pressure each time the catheter needs flushing, or by the volumetric pump administering the feed, constantly alarming. Perform a chest X-ray to look for kinking, flush with 10 mL heparinized saline, change dressing, instil 4 mL ethanol (clears lipid occlusion), urokinase 5000 IU in 1 mL (adult dose) will clear fibrin occlusion. If all these fail, the catheter will have to be removed and replaced, some centres advise the prophylactic use of low dose warfarin to prevent catheter occlusion.

Catheter damage
This occurs in long-term use due to repeated clamping and unclamping. The line must be clamped above the damaged portion and sterile gauze wrapped around the damaged part. Repair kits are available.

Extravasation
This occurs when the line displaces from the vessel or nutrient solutions infiltrate surrounding subcutaneous tissue. Remove the line immediately, assess damage to skin.

Weaning from PN
Improvement in the patient's condition and recovery of gastrointestinal function should prompt the institution of tube feeding or oral nutritional supplements and there should be a period of overlap. PN should be progressively weaned and stopped altogether

when the patient is able to tolerate the required amount of nutrients by the enteral or the oral route. Sudden stoppage of PN may result in a rebound hypoglycaemia and this can be prevented by the gradual withdrawal of PN.

Removal of lines

Lines can be removed at ward level as a sterile procedure with the patient lying flat in bed. Hickman lines have to be dissected out by a doctor skilled in the procedures but again this can be performed on the ward. All catheter tips should go to microbiology to enable audit of infection rates to be carried out.

Further reading

ASPEN Board of Directors and the Clinical Guidelines Task Force. Guidelines for the use of parenteral and enteral nutrition in adult and pediatric patients. *JPEN J Parenter Enteral Nutr* 2002; **26** (1 Suppl): 1SA–138SA.

National Collaborating Centre for Acute Care (2006). Nutrition Support in Adults: Oral Nutrition Support, Enteral Tube Feeding and Parenteral Nutrition. London: National Collaborating Centre for Acute Care. (http://www.rcseng.ac.uk/publications/docs/nutrition_support_guidelines.html).

National Patient Safety Agency. Advice to the NHS on reducing harm caused by the misplacement of nasogastric feeding tubes http://www.npsa.nhs.uk/health/display?contentId=3525.

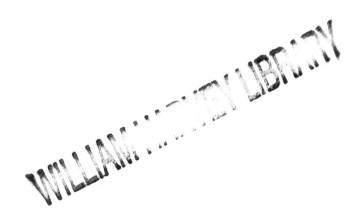

CHAPTER 7

Surgical Wounds

Alastair Simpson and Adam Brooks

OVERVIEW

- Define primary and secondary intention wound healing
- Be able to classify surgical site infection
- Recognize and use different types of wound dressing
- Identify the causes and correct management of abdominal wound dehiscence

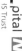

duction

Understanding the principles of wound healing and wound management is a fundamental aspect of surgical practice. Although surgeons are typically responsible for making wounds, much of the day-to-day postoperative care is performed by nurses, either on the ward or in the community, supported in complex cases by tissue viability nurse specialists. It is vital that these groups of health care professionals work together to achieve the best results for patients. Although primary closure is the goal in the vast majority of wounds and relatively little input is required, the problems posed by infection, wound breakdown and dehiscence require a significantly increased level of skilled management.

Wound healing

Healing by *primary intention* is the gold standard; this involves opposing fascial and epithelial edges to allow rapid healing with adequate tensile strength and minimal scarring (Figure 7.1).

If there is significant tissue loss or opposition of wound edges is not feasible then healing by *secondary intention* will occur. During this process granulation tissue is formed that contracts to reduce the wound area and allows epithelialization to proceed across its surface. Secondary intention wound healing is slower, producing a larger scar and results in only a thin protective layer with reduced strength (Figure 7.2).

ABC of Tubes, Drains, Lines and Frames. Edited by A. Brooks, P. Mahoney and B. Rowlands. © 2008 Blackwell Publishing, ISBN: 978-1-4051-6014-8.

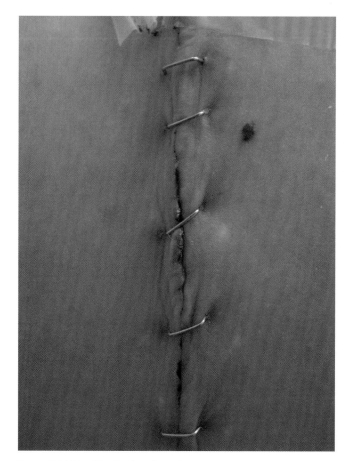

Figure 7.1 Wound healing by primary intention.

Wound infection

Surgical site infections (SSIs) are a constant risk associated with any surgical procedure. They represent a significant threat and are a persistent burden on health resources (Figure 7.3).

A simple classification system was developed in the USA in the 1960s to predict the degree of microbial contamination of different wounds (Table 7.1).

The rate of infection increases moving from the 'clean' to the 'dirty' groups, and prophylactic antibiotics should be provided to patients in the contaminated and dirty groups (Box 7.1; Figure 7.4).

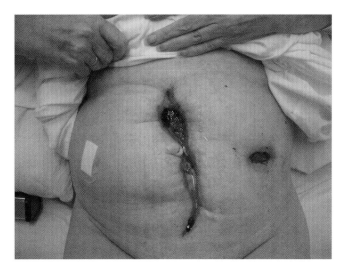

Figure 7.2 Wound healing by secondary intention.

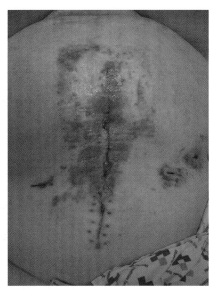

Figure 7.3 Superficial surgical wound infection.

Wound dressings

The aim of a wound dressing is to promote healing and reduce the risk of infection. The nature and site of the wound should determine the type of dressing used (Figure 7.5).

Wound dressings should possess a number of desirable properties. These vary depending on whether the wound being treated is moist, infected or a deep cavity. These properties are listed below:

- *Absorbancy* prevents the wound from becoming macerated. The bacterial permeability of a dressing should stop wounds from becoming infected by environmental pathogens and at the same time prevent spread of infection from a contaminated wound.
- *Adherence* of dressings to wounds is potentially damaging to the underlying healing process: during dressing changes granulation tissue may be damaged resulting in delayed healing.
- The *gas permeability* of dressings has been investigated without definite conclusion. Permeability to oxygen, carbon dioxide and water vapour is considered desirable.

Table 7.1 Classification of sugical site infections (SSIs). After Berard & Gandon (1964).

Classification	Criteria
Clean	Elective, not emergency, non-traumatic, primarily closed; no acute inflammation; no break in technique; respiratory, gastrointestinal, biliary and genitourinary tracts not entered
Clean-contaminated	Urgent or emergency case that is otherwise clean; elective opening of respiratory, gastrointestinal, biliary or genitourinary tract with minimal spillage (e.g. appendectomy) not encountering infected urine or bile; minor technique break
Contaminated	Non-purulent inflammation; gross spillage from gastrointestinal tract; entry into biliary or genitourinary tract in the presence of infected bile or urine; major break in technique; penetrating trauma <4 hours old; chronic open wounds to be grafted or covered
Dirty	Purulent inflammation (e.g. abscess); preoperative perforation of respiratory, gastrointestinal, biliary or genitourinary tract; penetrating trauma >4 hours old

Wounds heal best at near-normal body temperature. The physical and chemical properties of a dressing should not be detrimental to wound healing (Box 7.2).

Abdominal wound dehiscence

Abdominal wound dehiscence is the postoperative breakdown of the abdominal wound (Figure 7.6). Wound dehiscence can range from superficial dehiscence of the skin and subcutaneous tissues through to complete separation of the fascia. Post-laparotomy dehiscence can lead to e*visceration* (herniation) of abdominal contents (usually small bowel and omentum) outside of the abdominal cavity. Gauze soaked in normal saline should be applied to the eviscerated contents and the patient should be taken *urgently* to surgery.

Diagnosis

This is a clinical diagnosis and no studies are necessary for confirmation. Abdominal wall dehiscence may be a subtle clinical scenario whereby the patient senses a 'pop' when they move, cough or exert themselves. This is typically followed by a serous discharge from the wound. The frank evisceration of abdominal contents into the wound makes the diagnosis obvious.

Dehiscence occurs in up to 3% of patients following an open abdominal operation. There are multiple contributing factors for wound dehiscence listed in Table 7.2.

Technical features contributing to dehiscence include:

- Sutures too close;
- Sutures too far apart;
- Sutures too close to fascial edge;
- Wound closure under too much tension.

Polymicrobial infection is commonly involved in complete fascial dehiscence.

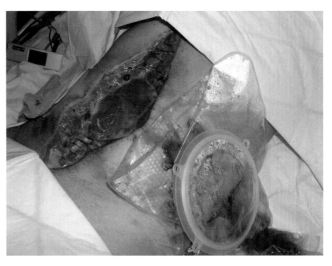

Figure 7.4 Deep surgical wound infection.

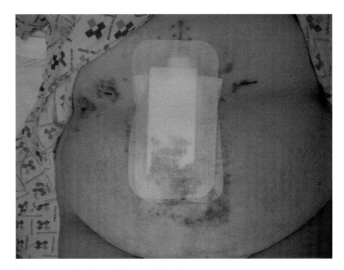

Figure 7.5 Typical surgical wound dressing.

Treatment
The goal of therapy following complete dehiscence is restoration of the abdominal wall. This is achieved by treating the underlying cause and creating a supportive environment (Box 7.3) in which wound healing can take place.

Evisceration:
• Initially cover wound with saline soaked gauze;
• Urgent surgical exploration (ensuring no intra-abdominal infection or anastomotic leak);
• Reduction of the contents;
• Re-closure of the abdominal wall;
• Necrotic fascia must be débrided and placement of retention sutures may be necessary.

Dehiscence without evisceration:
• Dressings to the wound and investigations to rule out intra-abdominal infection or further wound infection.

In the absence of evisceration, abdominal wall integrity can be restored by surgical closure of all or some of the abdominal wall layers or healing by secondary intention followed by split thickness skin graft over granulation tissue, component separation, prosthetic mesh placement and/or local or regional tissue flaps. Primary fascial closure should not be attempted after 7–10 days as the viscera are likely to have adhered to the anterior abdominal wall and the fascia will have retracted.

Retention sutures are large non-absorbable sutures placed through the fascia and skin at wide distances from the skin edge and are secured through a protective device to avoid skin necrosis should the abdominal wall become oedematous. Their use remains contentious as if they become excessively tight as the abdomen distends they can 'cheese-wire' through the skin or alternatively loose bowel can be trapped in a loop of retention suture.

Box 7.2 **Types of dressing**

Conventional dressing
- Consist of a non-adherent material covered by a more absorbent material such as gauze or wool. Kept in place by adhesive tape or bandage
- Indicated in wounds healing by primary intention, wounds with minimal infection risk and no slough or discharge
- Not suitable for moist wounds

Polyurethane dressings
- Semi-occlusive dressing, permeable to vapour and gases but not water or bacteria
- Can lead to accumulation of exudates or blood under the dressing, which is a disadvantage. However, studies suggest that moist wounds heal faster than dry ones
- These dressings also create an acidic environment, which in turn promotes angiogenesis, fibroblast proliferation and epidermal migration

Hydrocolloid dressings
- Consists of an adhesive hydrocolloid with a semi-occlusive foam and plastic film exterior
- The hydrocolloid absorbs exudates and forms a yellow liquefied gel
- Not suitable if exudate is too heavy
- Not suitable for dressing deep cavity wounds

Osmotic agents
- By means of osmosis slough is débrided from the wound and creates a moist environment
- Requires a second dressing. Honey is an old fashioned but effective example

Hydrogels
- An aqueous gel that contains a starch polymer matrix, which absorbs excess exudates but retains a moist environment. Used on dry, sloughy or necrotic wounds but not suitable if large volumes of exudate

Alginates
Require an outer dressing and if left too long hydrogels dry, become difficult to remove and can cause maceration of the surrounding skin

Foams
Have an inner hydrophilic area and an outer hydrophobic layer. Will conform to the shape of the wound. Require changing as the wound shrinks

Saline soaks
Favoured by many surgeons for rapid desloughing but requires regular changes (every 4–6 hours)

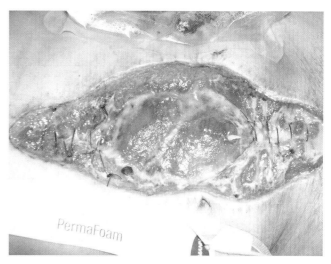

Figure 7.6 Abdominal wound dehiscence.

Table 7.2 Factors contributing to abdominal wound dehiscence.

Local factors	Regional factors	Systemic factors
Wound infection	Bowel oedema	Advanced age
Haematoma	Intrabdominal infection	Malnutrition
Seroma	Haemorrhage	Pulmonary disease
Imperfect surgical technique	Trauma	Renal failure Obesity Diabetes mellitus Steroid use Chemo/radiotherapy

Box 7.3 **Optimum conditions for wound healing**

- Uninfected
- Viable tissue without ischaemia
- No foreign bodies
- Near body temperature
- Optimum pH
- Atraumatic dressing changes

Diegelmann RF, Evans MC. Wound healing: an overview of acute, fibrotic and delayed healing. *Frontiers in Bioscience* 2004; **9**: 283–289.

Grey J, Harding K, eds. *ABC of Wounds*. 2006, Blackwell BMJ Books, Oxford.

Horan TC, Gaynes RP, Martone WJ, *et al*. CDC definitions of nosocomial surgical site infections, 1992: a modification of CDC definitions of surgical wound infections. *Infection Control and Hospital Epidemiology* 1992; **13**: m606–608.

Ysabel M, Bello MD, Tania J, Phillips MD. Recent advances i... *JAMA* 2000; **283**: 716–718.

Further reading

Berard F, Gandon J. Postoperative wound infections: the influence of ultraviolet arradiation of the operating room and of various other factors. *Annals of Surgery* 1964; **160**: 1–192.

CHAPTER 8

Surgical Drains

Sherif Awad, Alastair Simpson and Adam Brooks

OVERVIEW

• Reasons for placing drains include draining existing/potential collections, diversion of fluid, irrigation of a cavity and reducing seroma formation

• Use of drains must be balanced against increased risk of infection, damage to anastamoses and nearby structures, patient discomfort and subsequent reduced mobility

• Drains may be open or closed systems

• Daily drain (DRAIN) drill includes checking:

  • **D**aily volumes and type of fluid drained
  • **R**e-securing drain if loose or displaced
  • **A**dequate suction (if applicable)
  • **I**s it blocked, kinked or leaking
  • **N**eed for removal

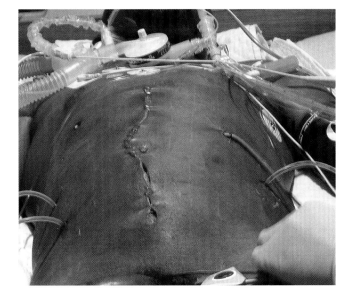

Figure 8.1 Patient with multiple drains.

Introduction

In general, surgical drains are inserted to:
• Drain existing collections (e.g. pus, blood, bile);
• Drain potential collections;
• Divert fluid away from a blockage or potential blockage;
• Allow irrigation of a cavity;
• Minimize dead space in a wound and prevent seroma formation;
• Decompress and allow escape of air (chest drain).

There is little evidence to support the widespread use of drains in surgery and their use remains controversial (Figure 8.1). Those in favour of their use argue that drains:
• Reduce the risk of infection;
• Prevent the accumulation of fluids such as blood, pus, bile or lymph;
• Allow early detection of anastomotic leaks; and
• Create tracts through which potential collections can drain.

The counter argument is that drains:
-          ·isk of infection;
             be caused by mechanical pressure or suction;

• May induce anastomotic leaks; and
• Much of the fluid drained is produced by the body in response to the presence of a foreign body.

Many different types of drain are employed to accomplish the objectives of drainage outlined above (Figure 8.2).

Open drains may drain into dressings or a wound drainage bag and by definition do not employ suction. Generally, open drains are not favoured as the collected fluid remains in contact with the skin causing maceration. The drained fluid may smell, there is a potential risk of increased infection and open drains can be painful to dress and change.

Closed drains drain into container systems which may be:
• *Active*: connected to a suction source creating a continuous pressure difference between the proximal and distal end of the drain and drawing fluid from inside to out; or
• *Passive*: dependent on gravity and the pressure differential between the body cavity and the exterior in order for fluids to be drained.

Examples of common drains and relative advantages and disadvantages are given in Box 8.1 (Figure 8.3).

ABC of Tubes, Drains, Lines and Frames. Edited by A. Brooks, P. Mahoney and B. Rowlands. © 2008 Blackwell Publishing, ISBN: 978-1-4051-6014-8.

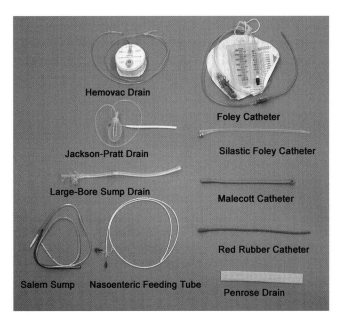

Figure 8.2 Different types of surgical drain.

Complications associated with the use of drains include:
- Complications of drain placement:
  Damage to nearby structures;
  Bleeding.
- Complications of drain residence:
  Leakage and skin excoriation;
  Infection via drain track;
  Damage to anastamosis (e.g. bowel);
  Retraction into the wound;
  Pain at drain site;
  Displacement/dislodgement of drain; and
  Decreased patient mobility.
- Complications after removal:
  Re-accumulation of collection after drain removal;
  Herniation at drain site (rare);
  Scar formation.

Management of drains

Drains should be cared for with the same degree of attention to detail that is required for all parts of the patient pathway. Drains should be inspected on a daily basis for the type of fluid and the quantity of content (24-hour totals). It is also important to ensure that the drainage system (from collection to bag) is patent and the drain is working correctly.

Daily drain drill

The following questions should be answered on a daily basis by the surgical team reviewing the patient:
1 Volume of fluid (24-hour total)
2 Type of fluid?
3 Blocked, kinked, leaking or displaced?
4 Adequately secured?

Box 8.1 **Drain types**

Open drains
Drain into a dressing or a bag open to the air, potentially increasing the risk of infection

Simple wicks
- Sterile cotton gauze inserted into a cavity or shallow wound
- Fluid will track along the material
- They require changing on a regular basis and may interfere with granulation tissue formation

Corrugated polythene drain
- Can be used for deep and superficial drainage
- Should be sutured in position
- Polyethylene induces very little tissue reaction

Yeates drain
- Similar in nature to the corrugated drain with similar indications but consists of a series of capillary tubes

Penrose drain
- Consists of a thin-walled rubber tube containing a fine length of gauze
- It is not as rigid as a corrugated or Yeates drain

Closed drains
Drain into an airtight system therefore risk of infection is reduced

Silastic tube drain
- Made from polymeric silicone and induce very little tissue reaction
- This allows rapid closure of any track following removal of the drain
- This system is useful for deep intraperitoneal drainage

Red rubber tube drain
- Causes intense tissue reaction therefore creates long-standing tract
- May be required to drain chronic abscess cavity, empyema or hepatic abscess

Suction drain (Jackson–Pratt, Redivac)
- It consists of a fine tube with many holes attached to an evacuation container
- Useful for the continuous drainage of blood post procedure, i.e. mastectomy or thyroidectomy
- When used intraperitoneal cavity can become blocked by omentum

Sump drain
- A suction tube with a double lumen
- An intake tube supplies air to the bottom of the main tube to which suction is applied. This allows fluid to be drained while the flow of air prevents blockage

5 Adequate suction (if suction drain; Figure 8.4)?
6 Ready for removal?

It is important to recognize whether blood, pus, faeces or haemoserous fluid is being drained (Figure 8.5) and *to recognize if this is the expected drainage fluid or not*. Quantity of fluid is not always a good guide to hidden pathology as large quantities of inflammatory exudates may be produced in normal healing mechanisms but it is

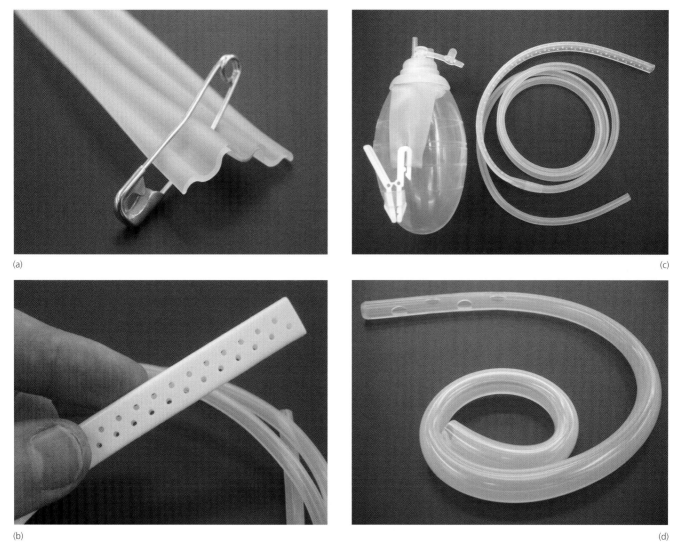

(a)

(b)

(c)

(d)

Figure 8.3 Surgical drains. (a) Corrugated drain. (b) Jackson–Pratt drain. (c) Grenade suction collection for a Jackson–Pratt drain. (d) Tube drain.

an essential measurement to be taken when considering the ongoing fluid requirements of a patient.

> **Never rely on absence of blood in a drain to reassure you that the patient is not bleeding**

One of the potential downfalls of drains is blockage. If the drain blocks or drains poorly because of thick pus then the drain can be flushed on a daily or twice daily basis with small volumes (20 mL) of normal saline. Blood and clot can also block drains and an empty drain can falsely reassure the unwary.

The drain tubing may kink or block especially where it enters a collection bag (Figure 8.6), securing sutures may become loose or cut through allowing the drain to 'fall out'. Checking these potential 'traps' is part of the daily drain drill.

Pitfalls/troubleshooting

- Drains that are collecting passively, i.e. not via a suction mechanism, must have the tube connecting the drain to the reservoir as well as the reservoir itself placed in a dependent position to the actual drain (Table 8.1).
- Ensure that the drain tubing is not compressed or kinked especially at the point that the drain enters the bag.

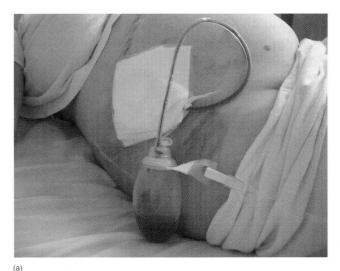

(a)

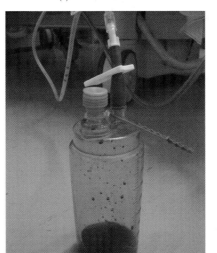

(b)

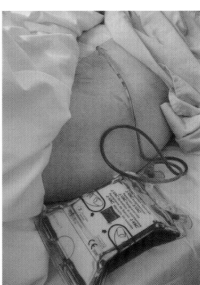

(c)

Figure 8.4 (a) Jackson–Pratt drain in use. (b) Redivac drain in use. (c) J-vac drain in use.

• Drains not adequately secured to the abdominal wall skin can mistakenly fall out or be pulled out during patient movement.
• Drain malfunction:
  The drain itself may slip out beyond the abdominal skin thus diminishing the efficacy of suction or straight drainage;
  Clogging of the drain perforations occurs secondary to clot or fibrinous material embedded in it. Many drains need to be 'stripped' frequently to prevent this from occurring;
Sump ports of sump drains may become clogged with effluent and prevent the airflow past the tip. Clearing the sump port will alleviate this.

Removal of drain

Absolute rules for the removal of drains do not exist but rather are based on experience and may vary from patient to patient and surgeon to surgeon. It is not a bad principle that the person who put the drain in should be the one to decide when it should come out. In general, the policy should be to remove drains at the earliest appropriate opportunity:
• If a drain has been placed to cover perioperative bleeding it can usually be removed after 24–48 hours;
• Drains to remove serous collections can usually be removed after 5 days;

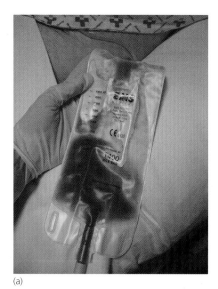
(a)

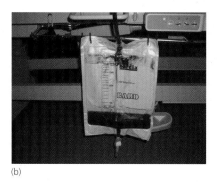
(b)

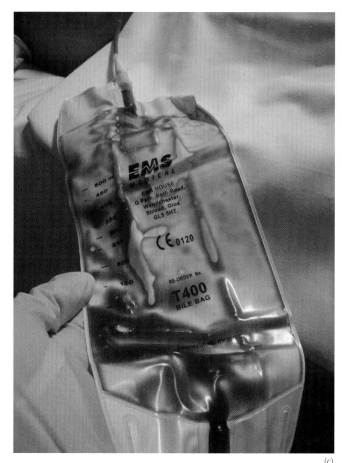
(c)

Figure 8.5 (a) Bile in a drain bag. (b) Blood in drain bag. (c) Haemoserous fluid in drain bag.

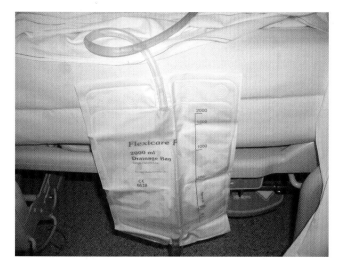

Figure 8.6 Kinked tubing blocking a drain bag.

Table 8.1 Troubleshooting drains.

Issue	Action
Thick inspisated pus/poor drainage	Twice daily drain flush with normal saline
Collection tubing kinked	Reposition/consider using a drain bag hanger
Collection bag empty	Check: Is bag not opened (therefore not working) No fluid to collect
Suction grenade drain full	Empty as this precludes any further drainage

which is essential to prevent subsequent biliary sepsis from bile leakage into the abdomen on removal;
• Prior to the removal of a suction drain, suction should be switched off and the drain monitored for 12–24 hours.

• Drains to remove infected material should be left until drainage becomes minimal and the patient's clinical condition has improved;
• T-tube drains to provide biliary drainage should be left for a minimum of 3–6 weeks. This will allow the formation of a tract,

CHAPTER 9

Hepatobiliary

Ian Beckingham, Sherif Awad, J. Edward Fitzgerald and Adam Brooks

OVERVIEW

- Patients with surgical drains are increasingly managed in the community and a thorough understanding of the types and roles of drains employed is crucial

- Percutaneous drainage is employed where endoscopic access and stenting has failed – these patients should be closely monitored for the resultant nutritional and metabolic sequelae of external loss of bile

- Internal drainage is prefered to external drainage

- Internal biliary drainage may be temporary to relieve jaundice or permanent in patients with unresectable tumours

Introduction

Hepato-pancreatico-biliary (HPB) surgery relies on a wide range of tubes, drains and stents to aid in the management of patients with these complex abdominal diseases. These can be placed at surgery (either open or laparoscopic), percutaneously (under radiological guidance) or endoscopically.

Patients with complex HPB conditions and postoperative complications may be managed by those outside the specialist team within local hospitals or in the community following an operation or endoscopic procedure. Understanding the role, functions and types of surgical drains and stents that are used within HPB surgery is crucial for all members of the multidisciplinary team involved in patient care.

Biliary system

T-tubes

Laparoscopic cholecystectomy, endoscopic retrograde cholangiopancreatography (ERCP) and magnetic resonance cholangiopancreatography (MRCP) have together reduced the incidence of common bile duct exploration and therefore the routine use of T-tubes (Figures 9.1 and 9.2). They are still used at open bile duct exploration and occasionally following laparoscopic

ABC of Tubes, Drains, Lines and Frames. Edited by A. Brooks, P. Mahoney and B. Rowlands. © 2008 Blackwell Publishing, ISBN: 978-1-4051-6014-8.

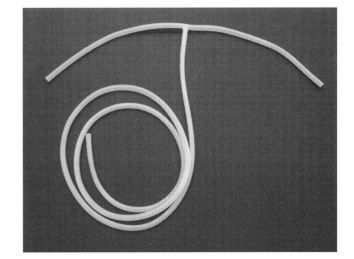

Figure 9.1 T-tube.

bile duct exploration to provide drainage of the biliary tract. Whereas normal drains are made of inert silastic material which does not excite a tissue reaction, T-tubes are made from rubber drains and have the opposite effect. Rubber excites an intense fibrotic reaction within the surrounding tissues, causing the formation of a tract around the drain. This may be useful in certain situations.

Indications and rationale for their use include:
- Following bile duct exploration – enables postoperative cholangiography and percutaneous extraction of retained stones.
- Protect bile duct repair or anastamosis – enables external bile drainage while the repair/anastamosis heals, thus reducing the occurrence of bile leak and biliary peritonitis.

The size of the T-tube should be correlated to the diameter of the common bile duct: 14 French gauge should be the smallest size used to enable subsequent interventional radiology.

The limbs of the T-tube are shortened to prevent proximal obstruction and distal entry into the duodenum, reducing the incidence of acute pancreatitis. Dividing the back wall of the T-tube may ease removal but at the expense of making interventional procedures more difficult. The T-tube is placed within the duct and repair fashioned ensuring the T-tube is not caught within the closing stitch.

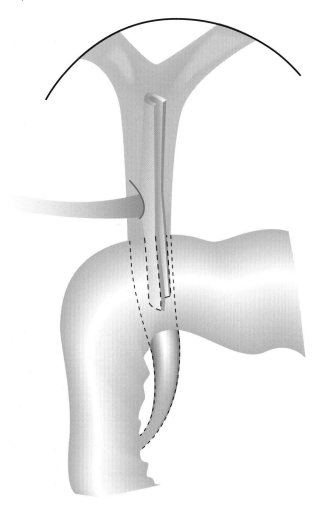

Figure 9.2 T-tube *in situ* within common bile duct (pancreas removed for clarity).

Postoperative management

It is important to ensure that bile flows freely through the drain after closure of the abdomen. Postoperatively, bile should drain freely into a bile bag and the volumes accurately recorded on a daily basis (see p. 45). The volumes drained vary but should decrease in time as normal flow into the duodenum (the path of least resistance) is established.

Potential postoperative problems that may be encountered are shown in Table 9.1. A T-tube cholangiogram can be performed at 2–3 days postoperatively. If this is normal, the T-tube can clamped and secured to the patient. Removal is delayed for 3–6 weeks to ensure that an adequate tract has formed, as early removal can be associated with a leak of bile into the abdomen. If the cholangiogram is abnormal, then subsequent management depends on the cause. If caused by continuing distal obstruction (e.g. duct stone) the patient is sent home and the cholangiogram repeated at 5–6 weeks. If intervention is necessary this may be performed by utilizing the fistula track formed by the T-tube.

Removal

Gentle traction should be all that is required for removal of the T-tube. If this fails, specialist advice should be sought.

Table 9.1 Potential T-tube complications.

Problem	Potential cause(s)	Investigation(s) of choice
Bile volumes drained remain high or increase	Persisting distal obstruction, blockage of distal limb of T-tube	T-tube cholangiogram
No drainage of bile	Blockage/dislodging of T-tube	T-tube cholangiogram
Leakage of bile around T-tube	Blockage/dislodging of T-tube	T-tube cholangiogram
Patient becomes unwell	Infection within the biliary system (cholangitis), biliary peritonitis	Baseline bloods and blood and bile cultures (and medical review)

External biliary drainage

Other methods of external biliary drainage include:
- Percutaneous transhepatic biliary drainage;
- Nasobiliary drainage.

Percutaneous transhepatic biliary drainage

Percutaneous drainage is usually employed for obstructions of the biliary tree where endoscopic access and stenting has failed. The procedure entails puncture of an intrahepatic bile duct with a fine needle under ultrasound guidance. Following successful visualization of the ductal system a drain is left *in situ* to allow external biliary drainage. Where possible the drain is placed across the stricture to provide internal and external drainage. While in most cases this achieves adequate biliary drainage, the inconvenience of an external percutaneous drain and the risk of infection and metabolic or nutritional sequelae through loss of bile, means that in all but a few select cases internal biliary drainage is preferred. This may be achieved at a second procedure with conversion of the external stent to a metal wall stent in malignant, intractable disease, or by a 'contained procedure' where a guidewire is passed through the internal/external drain and at ERCP a plastic stent is inserted using the duodenoscope (Figure 9.3).

Nasobiliary drainage

This is rarely used nowadays because of the problems of patient discomfort and dislodgement of the tube, and has been largely superseded by using internal drainage.

Internal biliary drainage

This entails the use of endoprosthetic stents placed either endoscopically or percutaneously.

Endoscopic biliary stenting is now an established technique, with a technical success rate of over 90%. The technique is employed at ERCP and is used to relieve biliary obstruction either by stones or malignant disease. Stents can be temporary (plastic) or permanent (metal) depending on the situation. The use of self-expanding metallic stents has been shown in randomized trials to have better long-term patency than traditional plastic stents. Furthermore,

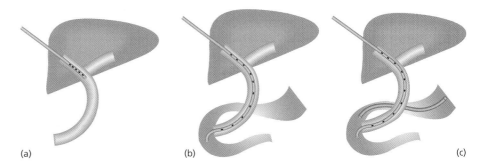

Figure 9.3 (a) External biliary drainage.
(b) Internal/external biliary drainage.
(c) Internalization of drainage at a combined
ERCP procedure (side viewing duodenoscope
shaded blue).

(a)   (b)   (c)

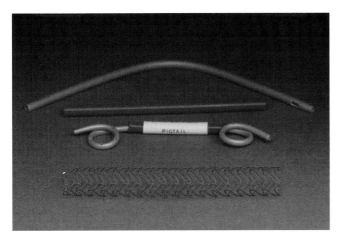

Figure 9.4 Endoprosthetic biliary stents. From top to bottom: plastic stent, stent straightener, pigtail stent and an expandable metal stent.

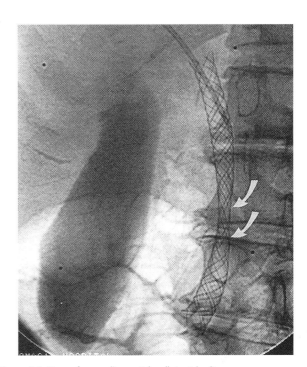

Figure 9.5 X-ray of expanding metal wall stent *in situ*.

metallic stents are less likely to migrate because of their incorporation within the wall of the duct. Complications relate to ERCP and the placement of a foreign body within the biliary tree and include pancreatitis (5%), perforation of the bile duct or duodenum (1%) and bleeding (1%). Later complications include stent migration (duodenal or biliary) and cholangitis resulting from stent blockage (Figure 9.4).

Transhepatic percutaneous stenting (PTC; see above) is an alternative when endoscopic stent placement fails or for hilar strictures where ERCP has a lower success rate than PTC. Potential complications include bleeding, cholangitis and biliary peritonitis (Figure 9.5).

Pancreatic drains

These are mainly employed in the management of pancreatic abscess/necrosis complicating severe acute pancreatitis. While discussion of the management of these complex conditions is beyond the scope of this chapter, the main principles and rationale for the use of drains are outlined.

The management of pancreatic necrosis and infected necrosis has evolved over the years and now entails a combination of several techniques including open laparostomy and planned re-exploration (Chapter 1), simple drainage of the surgically debrided cavity, closed lavage systems and the use of minimally invasive surgery.

The principles of management involve thorough debridement of all necrotic or infected tissue (often requiring repeat procedures)

balanced against limiting the physiological insult caused by long and complex surgery in these critically ill patients.

Following debridement, large diameter tube drains are used to allow either drainage of infected postoperative fluid collections (although drain occlusion is commonly caused by necrotic debris) or lavage of the cavity (the aim being continuous removal of necrotic material and debris).

Debate continues as to the best method of managing these patients and the choice between the different modalities of treatment depends on local expertise and experience.

Percutaneous cholecystostomy

This entails placing a drain percutaneously (through the skin) into the gallbladder to allow drainage of its contents (Figure 9.6).

The relative ease with which percutaneous cholecystostomy (PC) can be performed under ultrasound guidance makes it an ideal procedure in the critically ill patient whose condition precludes more aggressive intervention. Definitive treatment will, however, be required as PC acts only as a temporizing measure.

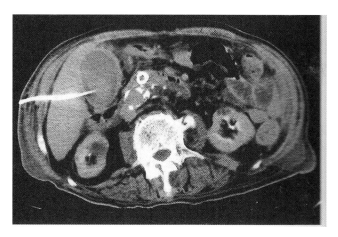

Figure 9.6 Computed tomography (CT) scan demonstrating a percutaneous cholecystostomy.

Indications for percutaneous drainage of the gallbladder include:
- Acalculus cholecystitis in critically ill patients;
- Acute calculus cholecystitis in patients too frail or ill to undergo cholecystectomy;
- Gallbladder empyema in patients who are high risk candidates for surgery.

Ideally, a self-retaining catheter with a locking loop should be used to reduce the risks of tube dislodgement.

Postoperative management

Drain fluid is sent for microbiological examination to determine appropriate antibiotic treatment. In acalculus cholecystitis improvement in the patient's condition can be expected in 50–80% of cases allowing removal of the drain and definitive therapy once the patient has recovered from their septic episode.

Further reading

Blumgart LH, Fong Y, eds. *Surgery of the Liver and Biliary Tract*, 3rd edn. W.B. Saunders, London, 2000.

Poston GJ, Blumgart L, eds. *Surgical Management of Hepatobiliary and Pancreatic Disorders.* Martin Dunitz, London, 2003.

CHAPTER 10

Stomas

Iain Anderson and Amanda Smith

OVERVIEW

- The support of a specialized stoma service is valuable in the care of these patients
- Stoma therapists provide the interface between primary and secondary care
- Preoperative siting prevents many late complications
- Most stomas issues are relatively easily managed

Introduction

Having a stoma poses significant physical and psychological challenges. While the care of the patient with a stoma has been transformed by the development of specialized stoma therapy services, many medical professionals remain uncertain about stomas. In fact, stomas are simply examined and usually straightforward to understand. Help is always available through the local surgical department or stoma therapy service.

Types

Typically, an ileostomy (Figure 10.1) has a 2-cm spout to prevent the more liquid effluent burning the skin, while a colostomy (Figure 10.2), with its more formed effluent, lies flush.

Either can be an *end* stoma (Figures 10.1 and 10.2) or a *loop* stoma (Figure 10.3). Often, the non-functioning lumen of a loop ileostomy is compressed by the spout and is largely hidden. A *mucous fistula* is a bowel stoma through which the stream of food and bile does not pass – usually because it is a distal end (Figure 10.4).

Common indications

Stomas can be made during a range of operations on the lower gastrointestinal tract. Some of the more common scenarios are described below.

A loop ileostomy is often created to temporarily defunction and protect a colorectal anastomosis made after excision of the upper

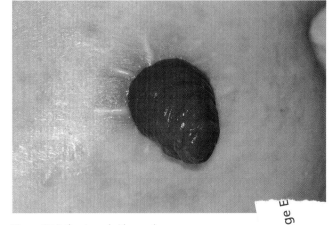

Figure 10.1 Ileostomy (with spout).

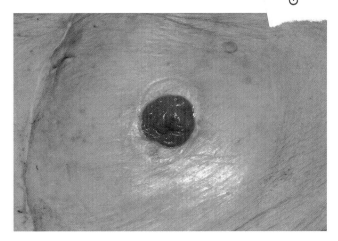

Figure 10.2 Colostomy (no spout).

rectum, typically for bowel cancer. This greatly diminishes the consequences of any leakage from the anastomosis in the postoperative period.

A Hartmann's operation (Figure 10.5) is still commonly carried out for perforated diverticulitis and obstructing or perforating cancers in critically ill patients. This leaves the patient with an end colostomy in the left iliac fossa.

Patients with severe acute colitis who require emergency colectomy usually have an end ileostomy in the right iliac fossa. The

ABC of Tubes, Drains, Lines and Frames. Edited by A. Brooks, P. Mahoney and B. Rowlands. © 2008 Blackwell Publishing, ISBN: 978-1-4051-6014-8.

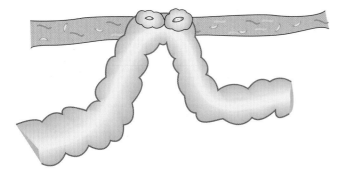

Figure 10.3 Loop colostomy.

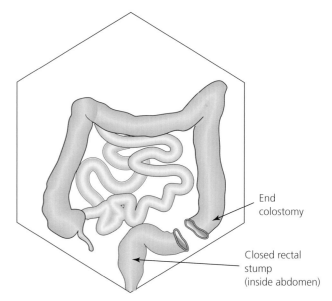

End colostomy

Closed rectal stump (inside abdomen)

Figure 10.5 Sigmoid resection, end colostomy, closure of rectal stump: Hartmann's procedure.

A colostomy will produce a semi-formed motion often working once or twice a day. The one or two-piece, usually sealed, bag is removed to change it. Some patients irrigate their colostomy in order to wash out the colon and prevent it working for a period. This allows them to wear a stoma cap – a bag with almost no capacity, which is almost invisible under light clothing.

Patients with a defunctioned rectum may continue to pass mucus plugs which can look alarmingly like stool. These can be difficult to pass and give an unpleasant feeling of rectal fullness: an enema provides relief.

Examining a stoma

Adequate examination requires removal of the stoma bag. Check that a spare is available. Stomas should be pink and healthy and the surrounding skin uninflamed. The stoma should accept a gloved and lubricated finger without significant discomfort. The little finger may be more appropriate for examining an ileostomy.

In the first few days after operation, the surgeon will wish to know whether the stoma has produced bowel contents (a small volume of thin serous blood-stained fluid may be seen before this) and whether it looks healthy. In creating an ileostomy, the bowel is everted and some degree of oedema is inevitable initially (Figure 10.6). Oedema can cause congestion of the mucosa but a dusky stoma may also be caused by bowel ischaemia: passing a flexible endoscope can assess the extent of duskiness. A full assessment of the patient is required to ensure that there is neither significant local ischaemia nor a more extensive problem with blood supply to the intestine requiring urgent intervention.

Complications of stoma creation

Creating a stoma leaves an inherent weakness in the abdominal wall and para-stomal hernia formation is extremely common, probably affecting 50% or more of stomas in time (Figure 10.7).

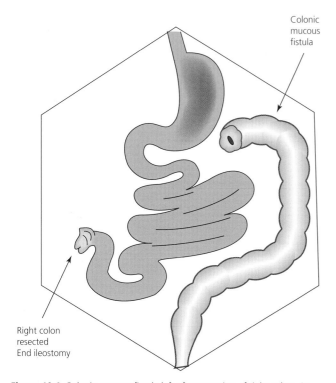

Colonic mucous fistula

Right colon resected End ileostomy

Figure 10.4 Colonic mucous fistula left after resection of right colon. An ileostomy is also present.

rectum is left in place and its upper end may also be brought to the skin as a rectal mucous fistula, akin to Fig. 10.4 but with only the rectum remaining.

Function

Stoma function varies significantly but an ileostomy typically produces 500–750 mL/day and most ileostomists use a drainable stoma bag that can be emptied (4–5 times per day) thereby reducing skin trauma. The bag is changed every 1–3 days. The further up the small intestine towards the stomach an ileostomy (or jejunostomy) sits, the greater its output will be. Dehydration is a risk, especially in warm weather and loperamide can help reduce the output. Output also depends on oral intake.

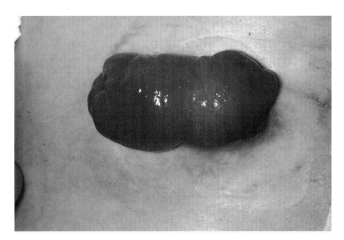

Figure 10.6 Oedematous ileostomy shortly after construction.

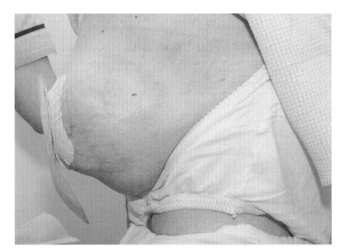

Figure 10.7 Large para-stomal hernia.

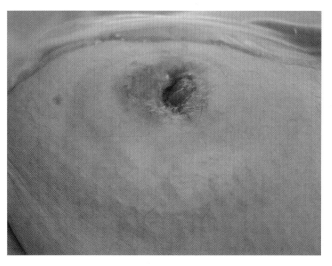

Figure 10.8 Retracted and stenosing colostomy.

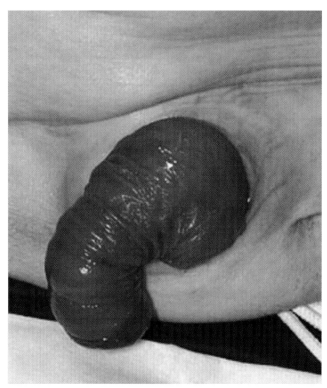

Figure 10.9 Prolapsing stoma.

Many para-stomal hernias are small and asymptomatic and are best left alone. When they enlarge, discomfort and difficulties with appliance fitting and clothing occur. Support belts and girdles can help but enlarging and symptomatic hernias should be repaired. This can be challenging and may involve re-siting the stoma or placement of a mesh. The incidence of recurrence is significant. Obstruction and strangulation of the bowel within a hernia is occasionally seen and is a surgical emergency.

Obesity or operative difficulty may lead to tension on the bowel resulting in retraction of the stoma or *ischaemic stricturing* (Figure 10.8). This can require emergency re-operation but lesser degrees of severity may be left alone in critically ill patients. A retracted stoma will have a puckered and uneven surround to which it is difficult to seal the stoma bag. The patient, with the help of their stoma therapist, can dilate lesser degrees of stenosis successfully. Laxatives may be required.

Stenosis of the skin can also occur later on, most often as a result of chronic skin inflammation. While this can be brought about by poor fitting of the stoma appliance, recurrence of any previous Crohn's disease should also be considered.

Conversely, stomas (typically loop colostomies) can pro-lapse themselves into the stoma bag, often enlarging alarmingly

(Figure 10.9). A surgical repair may be needed but early manual reduction by gentle sustained pressure is important especially if the prolapse is becoming oedematous.

Changes in stoma function require investigation. Constipation is particularly associated with sigmoid colostomies. If attention to diet and exercise is insufficient, oral laxatives or enemas via the stoma may be used. Ileostomists who complain of a non-function-ing stoma for 6 hours should seek medical advice. The patient may complain of pain, nausea and vomiting. Patients are advised to avoid solids, increase fluid intake, stop any anti-diarrheal medication and lie on their right side, massaging the peristomal area to dislodge

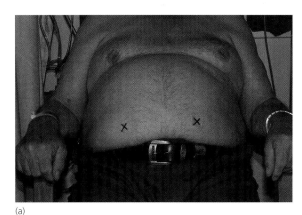

(a)

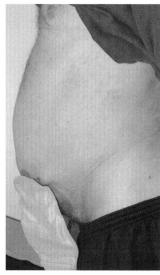

(b)

Figure 10.10 (a) Siting the stoma. (b) Poorly sited colostomy.

the usual food bolus blockage. Hospitalization may be necessary for the correction of dehydration and electrolyte imbalance. Once the problem has resolved the stoma therapist should ensure that the patient is aware of appropriate dietary restrictions.

Role of the stoma therapist and stoma siting

The stoma therapist provides a specialist interface between primary and secondary care, providing support in hospital before and after surgery and then in the community. Help is also available through information leaflets, telephone helplines and websites provided by national patient support groups and stoma product manufacturers (see further information).

Preoperatively, the stoma therapist and the patient agree on a visible and accessible stoma site (Figure 10.10). This minimizes any adverse impact on dressing, ability to manage the stoma and frequency of complications, especially appliance leakage. Information and support is given to the patient about prescription details concerning their appliance, nutritional advice, holidays, relationships, returning to work and social activities and prevention and detection of stoma complications. Patients can self-refer any time for further physical and psychological support; most stoma therapists offer open access via home visits or at outpatient clinics. There are many problems that can occur: most are simply addressed (Table 10.1).

Management of stoma and peristomal skin

Stomas vary. Initial postoperative oedema reduces after 4–6 weeks. However, the stoma also remodels itself throughout the patient's lifetime and it is essential that the aperture of the stoma bag

is altered accordingly, otherwise faecal dermatitis may occur (Figure 10.11). Water and cotton gauze is sufficient for cleaning faeces from peristomal skin and correcting the aperture usually resolves the problem within 72 hours.

Transient redness of the skin on removal of the appliance is not unusual and quickly disappears. Allergic contact dermatitis is rare. Peri-stomal rashes can be infective: culture and treat appropriately. Other pre-existing skin conditions can affect the peristomal skin but conventional treatments may interfere with adhesion of the bag.

The appearance of minimal blood on wiping clean the stoma surface is common. Surface bleeding may increase if the aperture of the bag is too tight. Bleeding from the stoma lumen proper needs further investigation, as this may indicate a recurrence of disease or infection.

Patients often report lumps and ulcers on their stomas. Granulations at the junction of skin and mucosa are not uncommon and seldom significant (Figure 10.12), although bleeding can affect adherence of the bag. Silver nitrate cautery can help. Traumatic ulcers can result from friction of the stoma bag or a trouser belt. Occasionally, ulcers on the stoma may indicate a recurrence of disease such as Crohn's.

If the patient complains about leaking bags, a complete assessment is undertaken of their stoma care technique, their nutritional status and discussion to identify any physical or psychological difficulties in coping with their stoma. There are very large ranges of stoma products and accessories that will assist even with the management of the most difficult stomas, but these should only be used under the direction of a stoma therapist (Figure 10.13).

Closing or reversing a stoma

Whether a stoma is temporary or permanent, reversal often depends more on the fitness of the patient and their desire to have it reversed

Table 10.1 Troubleshooting.

Problem	Cause/consider	Action
Bag leakage	Wrong size of aperture on stoma bag	Re-measure stoma and alter bag accordingly
	Poor patient technique	Refer to local ST for review and re-education
	Wrong type of bag for stoma type or output	Refer to ST. Guidance with diet and fluid intake and the use of medication as required
	Changes to patient's physique, i.e. weight loss/gain, skin creases or skin folds	Refer to ST for review of stoma bags: accessories may be required
	Unusual lumps (granulomas) on stoma affecting the adherence of the stoma bag	Refer to ST for advice: who may consider cauterising granulomas
	Parastomal hernia	Refer to ST for re-assessment of stoma bags and measuring of support belt/girdle
Sore peristomal skin	Leaking appliance causing faecal irritation	Re-measure stoma and alter bag accordingly
Rash on peristomal skin	Can be bacterial/fungal or pre-existing skin disease	Treat accordingly. Caution with creams/oils which will affect bag adherence
Constipation	Inadequate diet and fluid intake, reduced physical inactivity	Refer to ST. Review diet and fluid intake. Increase in physical activity
	Side effects of other regular medication	Change if possible. Use oral laxatives or enemas/suppositories via stoma
	Disease progression	Refer to specialist
Diarrhoea	Incorrect /inadequate diet	Refer to ST for advice
	Concurrent medication	Change if possible. Consider anti-diarrhoea/ rehydration medication
	Disease progression	Refer to specialist
	Faecal impaction for colostomist	See guidance for constipation
Non-functioning ileostomy	Partial or complete	Advise patient to avoid solids, increase fluid intake, stop any anti-diarrhoea medication. Seek specialist advice for correction of dehydration and electrolyte imbalance
	Obstruction may be dietary or mechanical	
Bleeding from stoma		
Mucosa	Cleaning stoma too vigorously	Spotting of blood is normal. Refer to ST for re-education
	Ill-fitting appliance	Re-measure stoma bag and alter accordingly
Lumen	Infection or disease progression	Treat and refer accordingly

ST, stoma therapist.

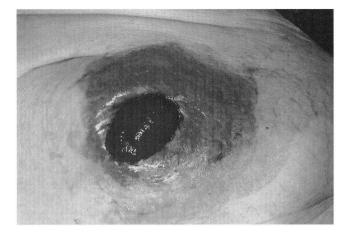

Figure 10.11 Peristomal dermatitis – often due to poor appliance fitting.

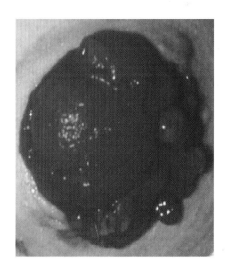

Figure 10.12 Granulations on ileostomy.

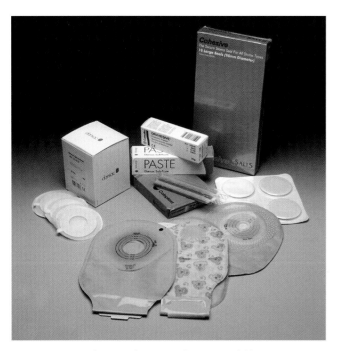

Figure 10.13 A wide range of stoma products are available.

than on the anatomy. The ease and success of reversal varies. A loop ileostomy is usually successfully reversed by means of a relatively modest operation. By contrast, reversing a Hartmann's operation traditionally requires a full laparotomy, is always a significant undertaking and can be a difficult operation. As many as 50% of the predominantly elderly patient group affected may decline the offer of further surgery.

Further information

The Urostomy Association
The Ileostomy and Internal Pouch Association
The Colostomy Association
Care of the Critically Ill Surgical Patient Course (CCrISP)

CHAPTER 11

Urology

Gurminder Mann

OVERVIEW

- Understand different types of bladder catheters
- Recognize indications for urethral catheterization
- Identify complications and rectify catheter complications
- Appreciate indications and use of ureteric stents
- Understand percutaneous access to the kidney

Introduction

Urologists are fortunate that the whole of the urinary tract can be accessed by artificial tubes of one form or another. This chapter describes methods and devices used for access to the urinary tract and describes some of the indications for such access.

Lower urinary tract (bladder and urethra)

Urinary catheters

Short-term (Foley) catheters are made of latex and can be left in place for up to 6 weeks before changing or removing. They are flexible and cheap, but are prone to infection. These catheters should be avoided in individuals with latex allergy or hypersensitivity (Box 11.1). Long-term catheters (e.g. silicone, Teflon) are typically left *in situ* for 3 months before changing (Figure 11.1).

Simple (in–out) or intermittent self-catheterization is performed to empty the bladder after which the catheter is removed.

Box 11.1 **Catheter types**

Single lumen (in–out)	–	Intermittent bladder emptying
Double lumen (Foley)	–	Prolonged bladder drainage
Triple lumen	–	Continuous irrigation after Urological surgery

ABC of Tubes, Drains, Lines and Frames. Edited by A. Brooks, P. Mahoney and B. Rowlands. © 2008 Blackwell Publishing, ISBN: 978-1-4051-6014-8.

In intermittent catheterization, a catheter is inserted through the urethra into the bladder to drain the urine completely. The catheter is then removed, cleaned and stored for use. This is a safe method of managing bladders that cannot empty because of neurogenic conditions such as spinal cord injury, spina bifida and multiple sclerosis. Improvement in bladder emptying reduces the risk of ascending urinary tract infection (UTI) and helps prevent renal failure in patients with spinal cord injury. This technique has transformed the lives of housebound patients and helped to preserve renal function in certain groups of patients.

Short-term catheterization using a self-retaining catheter is used for patients undergoing abdominal surgery or epidural anaesthesia. Catheterization allows surgery without hindrance by a full bladder and also allows monitoring of urine output during and after surgical procedures.

Acute urinary retention is distressing and may affect up to 10% of men in their seventies. It can be caused by a variety of conditions (Box 11.2). Immediate decompression using an indwelling catheter allows resolution of symptoms until the underlying condition can be addressed.

Long-term catheterization is an option for a variety of conditions and it is important that each patient is assessed individually. Incontinence (stress, urge, overflow, mixed or functional) that is refractory to conservative, pharmacological or surgical measures may be considered for long-term catheterization if intermittent catheterization is unsuitable. Bladder outlet obstruction that is not surgically correctable (i.e. patient not fit or unwilling) needs long-term bladder drainage. Permanent catheters can also be considered for terminally ill, immobile or severely impaired patients for comfort. Long-term catheters are easily exchanged in the community, occasionally by trained family members.

Catheter valves remove the need for drainage bags. They allow the bladder to fill naturally but rely on normal sensation so that a dextrous patient with good cognitive function can open the valve to empty the bladder via the catheter.

Supra-pubic catheterization (SPC) is performed under local or general anaesthetic by direct puncture of the bladder through the abdominal wall. It may be chosen as a matter of comfort or where there is urethral trauma. SPC is preferred by patients who are sexually active and by patients who are wheelchair-bound because of access advantages.

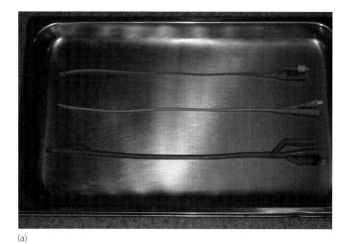
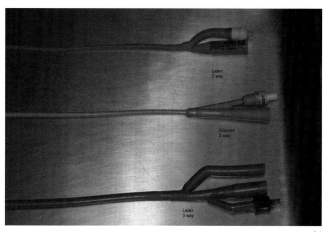

(a)   (b)

Figure 11.1 (a) Urinary catheters. (b) Top to bottom: short-term Foley catheter, long-term Foley catheter and a triple lumen catheter.

Box 11.2 **Causes of acute urinary retention**

Benign prostatic hyperplasia
Urinary infection
Cerebrovascular accident
Faecal impaction
Medication, e.g. tricyclic antidepressants, antispasmodics
Alcohol consumption

Upper urinary tract

Ureteric stents

Ureteric stents are thin flexible tubes that span the length of the ureter from the kidney to the bladder allowing urine to drain from the kidney. Ureters can become obstructed as a result of a variety of conditions; this obstruction can be acute or chronic in nature. A stent can be inserted to overcome obstruction and restore the flow of urine. In addition, stents can be used during and after urological surgery to provide a splint around which healing can occur, or be used to make ureters more easily identifiable during difficult surgical procedures (Boxes 11.3 and 11.4).

Stents are made from various materials such as polyurethane or silicone and can be left in place on a short-term basis (days to weeks) or on a longer term (weeks to months). They must be flexible, non-reactive, well-tolerated, non-migratory and be radio-opaque.

Stents can vary in length between 12 and 30 cm, depending on patient size, and typically have a diameter of 1.5–6 mm. One or both ends may form a natural coil (pigtail) to help retain it in position. These are often termed single-J or double-J (JJ) stents (Figure 11.2).

They are invariably placed under general anaesthetic in a retrograde fashion using a cystoscope. After identification of the correct ureteric orifice, a guidewire is passed under fluoroscopic control into the ureter up as far as the pelvis of the kidney. The guidewire provides a path for the hollow stent which is pushed forward until

Box 11.3 **Indications for stent insertion**

• Relieving ureteric obstruction (benign and malignant)
• Stone disease
  • Relief of obstruction
  • Aid passage of stone fragments after destruction
• Perioperative placement
  • Aid identification of ureter
  • Maintain ureteric lumen
• Management of urine leak
  • Iatrogenic leak
  • Leak caused by ureteric fistula

Box 11.4 **Causes of ureteric obstruction**

• Stones
• Tumours
• Blood clots
• Fungal infections
• Stricture disease
• Pelvic malignancy
• Prostatic disease
• Retroperitoneal disease

it reaches the renal pelvis. Satisfactory positioning of the stent can be checked using X-rays at which time the guidewire is pulled out from within the stent. At this time the pigtail loops reform (Figures 11.3 and 11.4).

If this retrograde method of stent insertion fails, an alternative approach would be antegrade stent insertion. This involves gaining access to the renal pelvis percutaneously (see below) and advancing a guidewire toward the bladder via this puncture site. The stent is then advanced over this guidewire in an analogous fashion.

Long-term stents need to be changed regularly (3–6 months) as they are prone to encrustation. Despite the evolution of modern materials patients may have irritative bladder symptoms, occasionally necessitating early stent removal. These symptoms are probably

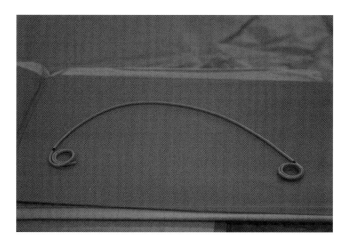

Figure 11.2 Ureteric JJ stent.

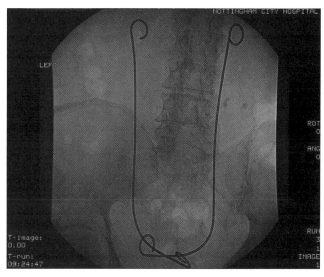

Figure 11.4 Ureteric JJ stent bilateral.

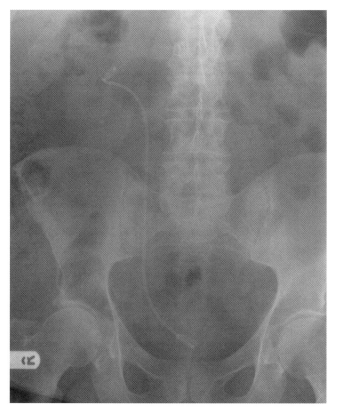

Figure 11.3 KUB Ureteric JJ stent unilateral.

brought about by the presence of the stent inside the bladder causing mechanical irritation. Infection and haematuria can also be caused by stents. Despite these complications normal activities can be carried out with a stent in place.

Removal of stents is usually carried out via a cystoscope. This procedure can easily be performed under local anaesthetic at which time the stent is visualized, grasped and removed intact.

Metal stents

Metal stents can be used to provide long-term drainage secondary to stricture disease or compression brought about by malignancy.

Metallic stents consisting of nickel-titanium (Nitinol) are thermo-sensitive. At cool temperatures the stent retains a compact form; once inserted into the body it expand to its original shape becoming softer and more elastic.

Stent coatings

Within a short time any prosthesis within the urinary tract is covered by a biofilm. This is a layer of host proteins, extracellular matrix and glycocalyx on the prosthesis surface. Bacteria can adhere and embed within the biofilm allowing protection from antibiotics. Different coatings have been developed for stents to reduce infection and the formation of biofilm. For example, Hydrogel coatings contain polyurethane polymers that swell with water which helps resist the formation of biofilm, encrustation and infection.

Drug eluting stents, used widely by cardiologists, are being developed for use in urology. Stents loaded with antimicrobials and dexamethasone are being currently assessed.

Percutaneous nephrostomy

A nephrostomy is a tract passing via the skin and body wall, through the renal tissue and ending in the renal pelvis. It can be used for a variety of purposes but commonly is used to drain urine when the ureter is obstructed and retrograde drainage (via the bladder) is not possible. Renal obstruction with superimposed infection is a urological emergency requiring prompt treatment. Rapid renal access using a nephrostomy can be life-saving and can be performed without the need for general anaesthesia which may be highly risky in such a septic patient. A nephrostomy can also provide access to the upper urinary tract for destruction or dissolution of renal calculi, antegrade radiological studies and stent placement as discussed above (Figures 11.5–11.8).

The nephrostomy is inserted using a combination of fluoroscopic and ultrasound guidance. A needle is inserted directly into the collecting system of the kidney through which a guidewire can

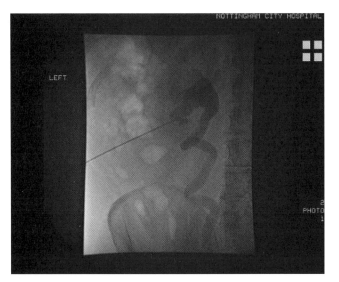

Figure 11.5 Percutaneous renal puncture prior to nephrostomy.

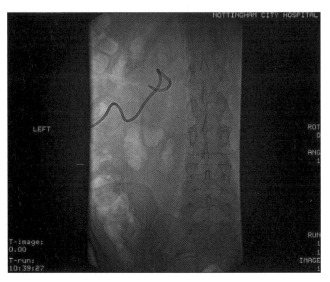

Figure 11.6 Nephrostomy plain film.

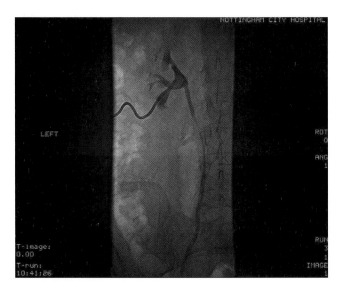

Figure 11.7 Nephrostomy contrast film.

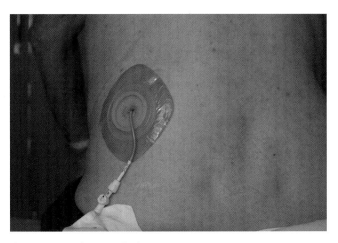

Figure 11.8 Nephrostomy *in situ*.

Table 11.1 Troubleshooting catheters.

Symptom	Action
Blocked catheter	Flush catheter; replace if unable to restore drainage
Urinary infection with catheter *in situ*	Treat infection if systemically unwell. NB all catheters will cause bacteriuria
Haematuria	Encourage oral fluid intake if bleeding not severe
Haematuria blocked catheter	Referral to urologist for bladder irrigation
Traumatic catheterization	Encourage oral fluid intake; may require antibiotics
Bladder pain from catheter	Consider oral anticholinergic therapy

be inserted. The tract can be widened using a selection of dilators and once established a hollow flexible tube can be inserted into the collecting system to drain urine. This tube can be altered once in position so that a pigtail is formed to retain the nephrostomy tube in place. Alternatively, a nephrostomy can be placed at the time of open surgery to obtain the same outcome.

A nephrostomy can be a short-term measure until the underlying obstruction is diagnosed and dealt with allowing subsequent removal of the nephrostomy. In other cases, nephrostomies can be used as a long-term solution if the underlying condition is non-correctable. Long-term nephrostomies can be exchanged.

Urostomy/ileal conduit

A few people who have cancer of the bladder will have a complete cystectomy and diversion of the urine flow into a section of the small bowel which is diverted to the abdominal surface to form a urostomy. These stomas are very similar to manage to colorectal stomas and further general information can be found in Chapter 10.

Further reading

Blandy J. *Lecture Notes on Urology*, 5th edn. Blackwell Science, Oxford, 1998.

Ellsworth P, Caldamone A. *Little Black Book of Urology*. Jones and Bartlett, 2007.

McLoughlin J, O'Boyle PJ, *et al. Top Tips in Urology*. Blackwell Science, Oxford; Cambridge, MA, 1995.

Tanagho EA. *Smith's General Urology*, 17th edn. McGraw-Hill Medical, New York, 2008.

Weiss RM, George NJR, O'Reilly PH. *Comprehensive Urology*. Mosby, London, 2001.

CHAPTER 12

Central Nervous System

Jerard Ross, Dawn Williams and Neil Buxton

OVERVIEW

- CNS drains and lines are usually managed within the hospital; however, specialists may not always be immediately available
- CNS drains and lines are usually inserted for monitoring the intracranial pressure (ICP) or cerebrospinal fluid (CSF) drainage
- CSF drains can block either due to collapse of the ventricles, ingress of choroid plexus or debris, infection or displacement
- Specialist advice should always be sought when troubleshooting these lines

Introduction

There are a number of situations in which lines and drains may be placed within the confines of the cranium and spine to aid management of patients with neurological illness. These are usually managed within a hospital environment with specialists on site but perhaps not immediately to hand.

The majority are aimed at monitoring the intracranial pressure (ICP) and less frequently externalizing cerebrospinal fluid (CSF) drainage; in some situations these can be complementary functions (Box 12.1).

Box 12.1 **Abbreviations**

ICP	Intracranial pressure
CPP	Cerebral perfusion pressure
CSF	Cerebrospinal fluid
CBF	Cerebral blood flow
MAP	Mean arterial pressure (diastolic pressure + one-third of the pulse pressure)
GCS	Glasgow Coma Scale

ABC of Tubes, Drains, Lines and Frames. Edited by A. Brooks, P. Mahoney and B. Rowlands. © 2008 Blackwell Publishing, ISBN: 978-1-4051-6014-8.

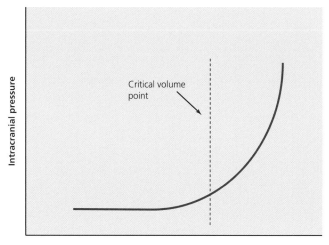

Figure 12.1 Pressure–volume curve. As the intracranial volume rises initially the pressure remains static as cerebrospinal fluid (CSF) and blood are displaced. At a critical point on the curve the compensatory reserve has been exhausted and in the brain a small rise in volume results in a significant rise in pressure.

Physiology of intracranial pressure

The cranial cavity (average volume 1500 mL) is, effectively, a closed box with one exit, i.e. the foramen magnum. It normally has relatively fixed contents of brain (1300 mL), CSF (75 mL) and blood in the venous and arterial compartments. Additional volumes in this closed box will eventually result in raised ICP (Figure 12.1), and if the pressure is high enough the brain will herniate (Figure 12.2) out of the cranium through the foramen magnum and the patient will die. This is known as the Monro–Kellie doctrine.

The ICP rises to potentially critical levels when conditions such as blood clots, brain swelling or excess intracranial CSF (in hydrocephalus) occur. Elevated ICP may impede cerebral blood flow (CBF) and result in critical brain ischaemia. This is important after brain trauma when the brain loses its intrinsic capacity to 'autoregulate' CBF and becomes 'pressure passive' (Figure 12.3). Therefore, after trauma the brain relies on an adequate blood pressure for perfusion, giving rise to the concept of the cerebral perfusion pressure (CPP). Measurement of the ICP allows calculation of the CPP from the mean arterial pressure (MAP):

$$CPP = MAP - ICP$$

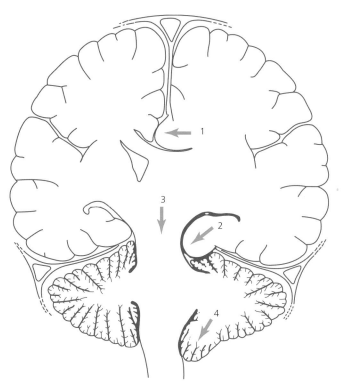

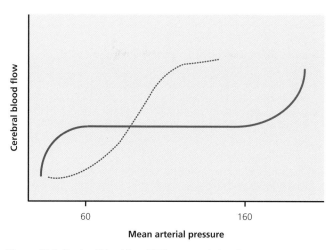

Figure 12.2 Patterns of brain herniation. (1) Cingulate herniation under the falx. (2) Uncal herniation through the tentorial incisura. (3) Central transtentorial herniation through the incisoral notch. (4) Cerebellar tonsillar herniation through the foramen magnum. The response of the brain to pathologically elevated intracranial pressure (ICP) is brain herniation. The most clinically important herniations being uncal herniation (2) (dilated ipsilateral pupil from IIIrd nerve compression, reduced consciousness and contralateral hemiparesis from cerebral peduncle compression) and transtentorial herniation (4) (bradycardia and hypertension and subsequently death).

Figure 12.3 Cerebral blood flow (CBF) autoregulation. Between mean arterial pressure (MAP) of 60 and 160 mmHg CBF remains static. The dotted line indicates CBF after loss of autoregulation when the blood flow is directly related to the cerebral perfusion pressure (CPP) and hence the MAP.

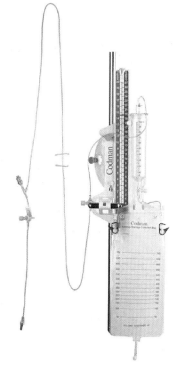

Figure 12.4 External ventricular drainage collection set. (Photo courtesy of Codman.)

Measurement of ICP and management of both the ICP and CPP have become central to modern care of the brain injured patient.

How do we monitor intracranial pressure?

The 'gold standard' for ICP monitoring is a catheter introduced into the lateral ventricle of the brain and coupled to an external pressure transducer. This is referred to as an external ventricular drain (EVD) and has the added advantage of allowing withdrawal of CSF to lower raised ICP directly (Figure 12.4). EVDs may be complicated by infection, blockage and migration. EVDs may be difficult to insert into the compressed lateral ventricles of a swollen brain.

More commonly, ICP is measured with fibreoptic pressure transducers placed in the brain parenchyma directly although they may be placed in the subdural space or intraventricularly. They produce accurate measurements of ICP and allow measurement of trends in ICP over time. The intraventricular pressure and the intraparenchymal pressure are generally equivalent. Commonly used types include the Codman microsensor (Johnson and Johnson), and the Camino ICP Bolt (Camino Labs) (Figure 12.5; Box 12.2).

ICP waveform

Although the term 'normal ICP' is discussed frequently, in reality ICP varies second to second and minute to minute and what is being described is the time averaged mean ICP. The basic ICP waveform (Figure 12.6) consists of three characteristic peaks temporally related to the arterial pressure waveform. There are, in addition, slower fluctuations related to the respiratory pattern. The central venous pressure is also important as there are no valves between the intrathoracic

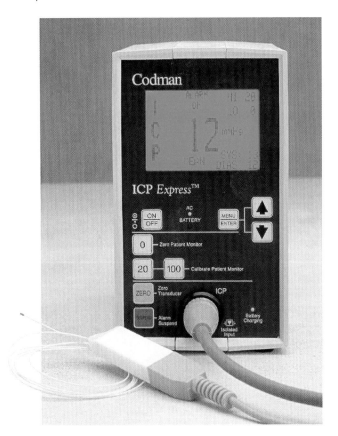

Figure 12.5 Intracranial pressure (ICP) monitor. (Photo courtesy of Codman.)

Box 12.2 **Intracranial pressure**

Normal supine adult ICP: 7–15 mmHg
ICP lower in infants and children
ICP lower when standing
ICP treatment threshold (adults): 20–25 mmHg
CPP = MAP – ICP
CPP ≥ 60 mmHg

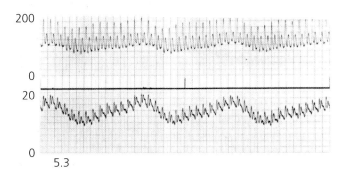

Figure 12.6 Comparison of the arterial pressure waveform (upper) and the intracranial pressure (ICP) waveform (lower). The three peaks of the ICP waveform are demonstrated clearly and the slower variation of the baseline seen in more prolonged monitoring is clear.

veins and the dural sinuses and as such pressure changes are transmitted directly to the intracranial cavity via the venous system. This is seen in healthy individuals performing a Valsalva manoeuvre (e.g. coughing), which results in marked but transient rises in ICP.

How is ICP monitoring used in practice?

ICP monitoring is not a treatment but rather is used as a guide for therapy to optimize the intracranial environment to improve outcome (Box 12.3). Sustained high ICP and/or low CPP is associated with excess mortality and poor outcome after severe head injury. ICP monitoring should be incorporated into protocols to allow a graduated introduction of therapy to optimize ICP. A staged approach to the report of an elevated ICP in a head injured ITU patient is outlined in Box 12.4.

Box 12.3 **Indications for ICP monitoring**

In trauma
Coma* and abnormal computed tomography (CT) scan
Coma after resuscitation with normal scan and any of: age >40 years, hypotension (systolic <90 mmHg), not localizing to painful stimuli
After removal of traumatic mass lesion
Multiply injured patient with altered level of consciousness who cannot be monitored clinically (e.g. serial GCS)
* (GCS ≤ 8) after resuscitation

In other settings
Coma from non-traumatic pathologies (meningitis, hepatic encephalopathy)
Diagnosis of raised ICP in CSF flow disorders and craniosynostosis

Box 12.4 **What should I do with an elevated ICP in a head injured patient in ICU?**

Stage 1
• Check the monitor is working
• Check the patient's pupils
• Make sure the head is not excessively rotated
• Make sure the venous outflow is not obstructed (e.g. ties on the endotracheal tube excessively tight, poorly fitted cervical orthosis)
• Elevate the head of the bed to 10–15°
• Check arterial blood gases are optimized (PaO_2 ≥ 11 kPa, $PaCO_2$ ≈ 4.5 kPa)
• Check patient is not febrile
• Check patient appropriately sedated and if necessary paralysed with muscle relaxant

Stage 2
• Osmotherapy (0.5 g/kg mannitol i.v. bolus/hypertonic saline)
• Vasoactive drugs (e.g. norepinephrine) to support CPP
• Optimize $PaCO_2$ 4–4.5 kPa
• Consider re-scanning to rule out surgical lesion

Stage 3
• Thiopental coma with electroencephalography (EEG) monitoring
• Insert external ventricular drain (EVD) and drain CSF
• Decompressive craniectomy

What are the complications of ICP monitoring?

Complications depend on the type of monitor employed and duration of monitoring. Infection is a significant complication of EVDs, as is haemorrhage, blockage and displacement. The rate of infection is less with intraparenchymal monitors and they cannot become blocked. However, there is a risk of drift in measurement over time, although this is less of a problem with the modern systems. Like EVDs they can become displaced.

Cerebrospinal fluid drains

To understand the use of CSF drains it is necessary to understand the basics of CSF physiology. CSF is produced in the cerebral ventricles, primarily by a process of active secretion by the choroid plexus and to a lesser extent from brain metabolism. It is produced at a rate of 0.33–0.35 mL/min^{-1}, i.e. around 500 mL/day.

External ventricular drainage can be used to monitor the ICP in the acutely brain injured patient; there are, in addition, other indications for CSF drainage (Box 12.5). In addition to drainage from the cerebral ventricles, CSF can also be safely drained from the lumbar theca in circumstances when the ICP is not raised by an intracranial mass.

When caring for a patient with an external CSF drain it is important to document hourly the patency of the drain, the volume in that hour and the running total of drainage as well as the patient's conscious level. CSF volumes drained from the cranial cavity should be replaced intravenously/enterically to avoid significant volume depletion; this is of particular importance in infants who can become significantly volume depleted from CSF drains.

CSF drains frequently block either as a result of collapse of the ventricles secondary to overdrainage, to ingress of choroid plexus or debris, because of infection or displacement. There is a role for flushing of drains to remove blockage, but this should be performed by those experienced in the management of drains and their complications and ideally by someone who can replace the drain if need be (i.e. a neurosurgeon).

The EVD works by gravity, the chamber height determining the ICP that must be reached before CSF drainage occurs: the higher the chamber, the greater the pressure. The patient with an EVD requires frequent monitoring by nursing staf (Box 12.6).

Box 12.5 Indications for continuous external CSF drainage

- Acute hydrocephalus (e.g. congenital or acquired causes)
- Raised ICP after trauma
- CSF fistulae (iatrogenic, traumatic or spontaneous)
- Diagnostic tests (e.g. lumbar drainage and CSF dynamics in normal pressure hydrocephalus)
- To allow instillation of therapeutic agents (e.g. antibiotics, chemotherapeutic agents)

Box 12.6 Important parameters to monitor in external ventricular drains

- Neuro-observations (GCS, pupillary light response, limb movements, temperature, pulse, blood pressure)
- Positioning of the collection chamber
- Appropriate levelling at the zero reference
- Patency of the catheter (is the CSF meniscus oscillating?)
- Amount of drainage
- Colour of CSF
- Exit site/pillow for signs of leakage

Box 12.7 Symptoms and signs of raised ICP

In the infant and young child

- Irritable, impaired level of consciousness, vomiting, failure to thrive, poor feeding, developmental delay
- Increased head circumference, tense anterior fontanelle, dilated scalp veins, 'setting sun' sign (the combination of upper eyelid retraction and failure of up-gaze)

In the older child and adult

- Headache, vomiting, drowsiness, diplopia, worsened seizure control
- Impaired consciousness and coma, impaired up-gaze, papilloedema
- Hydrocephalus of more gradual onset may cause dementia, gait ataxia and urinary incontinence (frequently seen in 'normal pressure' hydrocephalus)

Hydrocephalus

Hydrocephalus is an excess of intracranial CSF resulting in raised ICP. The aetiology is varied and includes both congenital and acquired causes (e.g. meningitis, haemorrhage) but all can result in symptoms and signs of raised ICP (Box 12.7), which vary depending on whether or not the cranial sutures are fused.

External CSF drainage is frequently employed in the immediate management of hydrocephalus and its complications. In an emergency, especially in the acutely ill person presenting *de novo* with hydrocephalus, gaining access to the cerebral ventricles to control pressure and examine the CSF is vital. This is most easily obtained through placement of an EVD or, alternatively, insertion of a ventricular access device which is placed in an identical fashion but accessed through the skin with a needle rather than being tunnelled extracranially.

Treatment options for hydrocephalus include insertion of a ventriculoperitoneal shunt, a tunnelled subcutaneous catheter and valve system carrying CSF from the ventricle to the peritoneal cavity. Most shunts have a built in CSF reservoir to allow emergency access to the CSF for drainage if the shunt becomes blocked and assessment of the CSF if there are signs of infection (Figures 12.7 and 12.8).

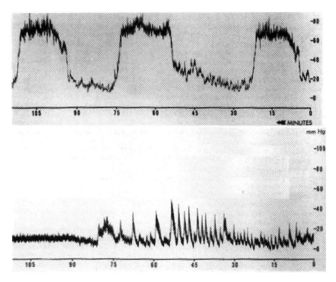

Figure 12.7 Intracranial pressure (ICP) traces. The top trace shows classic plateau waves of high pressure while the lower trace shows B waves. Both are pathological, although the aetiology is unclear.

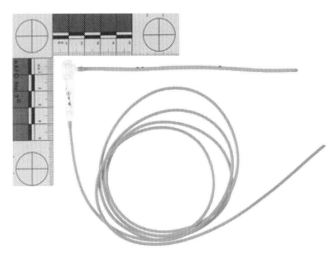

Figure 12.8 Ventriculoperitoneal (VP) shunt. Antibiotic impregnated VP shunt showing straight ventricular catheter, valve and reservoir and coiled peritoneal catheter.

Box 12.8 **Causes of CSF fistulae**

- Skull base trauma (CSF rhinorrhoea and/or otorrhoea)
- Postoperative, especially after skull base surgery (e.g. vestibular schwannoma resection, trans-sphenoidal pituitary surgery) and posterior fossa surgery
- Rarely spontaneous

In CSF infection the shunt may be externalized anywhere along its length to allow control of drainage and instillation of antibiotics. Similarly, if there is intraperitoneal sepsis in someone with a ventriculoperitoneal shunt, either primary or secondary to the shunt

itself, then the shunt should be externalized; however, if the shunt is happened upon during an intraperitoneal procedure for another pathology it is best left alone.

Lumbar drains

Lumbar drainage is not suitable for all types of hydrocephalus although it can be safely employed for hydrocephalus not secondary to intraventricular obstruction, i.e. those in whom there is free communication between the intraventricular CSF and CSF in the subarachnoid spaces (*syn.* communicating hydrocephalus). Lumbar drainage is frequently employed when a CSF fistula is present (Box 12.8).

Miscellaneous drains and wires

Wound drains

Closed wound drains are used variably by neurosurgeons and there is no class 1 evidence to support or refute their deployment. In intracranial surgery they are generally placed in the subgaleal space, often with gentle suction from a vacuum system. In extradural spinal surgery drains are sometimes left in the extradural space to prevent postoperative haematomas.

Cervical spine orthoses, frames and traction

In patients with potential or actual cervical spine instability external devices may have to be fitted to reduce fractures/subluxation or maintain alignment. This is achieved by traction, e.g. with Gardener–Wells tongs. These can be applied under local anaesthetic directly into the skull and the amount of weight attached is usually in the order of 1 kg per motion segment (i.e. C5/6 subluxation would require at least 5 kg of traction). Once appropriate alignment is obtained, position may be maintained by bony fusion or fixation and usually by a combination of both.

Orthoses are often used to limit movement of the cervical spine and can be applied in non-specialist settings. There are many different types, categorized into collars, poster-type orthoses and halo orthoses. Collars include the soft collar (having no useful function in terms of limiting cervical spine movement), the rigid Aspen and the Philadelphia collars. The Aspen is frequently used by emergency services and usefully limits flexion–extension movements having little effect on rotation or lateral flexion. The Philadelphia collar has similar efficacy but is more comfortable to wear for prolonged periods. Poster-type orthoses include the sterno-occipital mandibular immobilization (SOMI) brace which limits flexion–extension movements to a greater degree than rigid collars. Halo vests are the most reliable method of controlling cervical spine motion especially in the upper segments to C3. Halo braces fix the skull rigidly to a padded inflexible jacket, can be applied under local anaesthetic and are magnetic resonance imaging (MRI) compatible. The patient remains in this for a period of usually 12 weeks.

Further reading

Chambers IR, Jones PA, Lo TY, *et al.* Critical thresholds of intracranial pressure and cerebral perfusion pressure related to age in paediatric head injury. *Journal of Neurology, Neurosurgery, and Psychiatry* 2006; **77**: 234–240.

Czosnyka M, Pickard JD. Monitoring and interpretation of intracranial pressure. *Journal of Neurology, Neurosurgery, and Psychiatry* 2004; **75**: 813–821.

Girling KJ, Riley B. Neurological critical care. In: Brooks AJ, Girling K, Riley B, Rowlands BJ, eds. *Critical Care for Postgraduate Trainees.* Arnold, London, 2005.

Winn R, ed. *Youmans Neurological Surgery*, 5th edn. Elsevier, 2004.

CHAPTER 13

Frames, Pins and Plaster

Ian Pallister

OVERVIEW

- *The basics of fracture care*: reduce, hold and rehabilitate
- *Principles of external fixation*: temporary spanning fixation or definitive treatment
- *Pin site care*: how to tackle everyday problems
- *Infection*: how to spot a looming disaster and head it off
- *Compartment syndrome*: the importance of recognizing it, and the urgency of fasciotomy, its one and only treatment

Introduction

Fracture care is centered on the three basic principles of reduce, hold and rehabilitate (Box 13.1). Plaster of Paris and external fixator frames are widely used in acute fracture care for both immediate 'first aid' splintage and also for definitive care. All forms of effective treatment carry risk if they are applied improperly or not cared for attentively. A firm grasp of the basics of why a particular method of treatment has been adopted goes a long way to preparing one to care for that patient and foresee and forestall any associated problems.

The severity of an injury relates to its mechanism. Although much attention focuses upon the fracture, it is usually the associated soft tissue trauma that will determine how well a patient ultimately recovers once the fracture is united. Crush injuries, high energy transfer trauma (e.g. motor vehicle collisions and direct blows in contact sports) and open fractures can be associated with severe soft tissue trauma, the extent of which (or zone of injury) and its severity may not always be apparent at presentation. Once an acute

Box 13.1 **Principles of fracture care**

Reduce
Hold
Rehabilitate

ABC of Tubes, Drains, Lines and Frames. Edited by A. Brooks, P. Mahoney and B. Rowlands. © 2008 Blackwell Publishing, ISBN: 978-1-4051-6014-8.

fracture is immobilized, whether in plaster of Paris, a frame or with internal fixation, then the pain should steadily diminish with the passage of time. If the pain worsens, this is very sinister and can herald the development of *compartment syndrome*, or infection, both of which are catastrophic if overlooked.

External fixators and frames

External fixators are essentially scaffolds attached to the bone of injured limbs to maintain the reduction of the fracture. The bones themselves may be secured to the frame by stout metal pins with a threaded screw-like end fixed in the bone (threaded half-pins) or, alternatively, with fine wires that transfix the bone and are then tensioned before being secured to a circular ring on the frame, in the same manner as a spoke in a bicycle wheel. Broadly speaking, frames can be applied either as simple temporary spanning frames in damage control surgery, or in more complex configurations that can be used for definitive care (Figures 13.1 and 13.2).

Experience dating back to the First World War has shown the benefits of early fracture immobilization. However, in the 1990s it

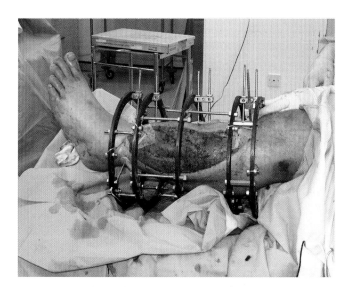

Figure 13.1 Ilizarov frame. Here the frame has been applied for definitive limb salvage purposes and the healed split skin grafted lateral fasciotomy wound can be seen.

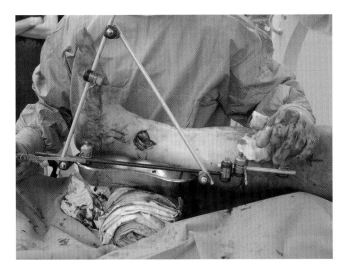

Figure 13.2 External fixator. A temporary spanning fixator applied for an open complex articular fracture of the distal tibia (plafond fracture). Near–far fixation is achieved with two pins in the foot (one in the first metatarsal base and the other transfixing the canlcaneum) and proximally with pins in the tibia away from the zone of injury. Note how the view of the wound is clear and no metalwork will cast a shadow over the zone of injury at computed tomography (CT) scanning.

> Box 13.2 **Correctly executed external fixation**
>
> Correctly executed spanning external fixation should:
> - Be rapid and simple to apply
> - Provide satisfactory *temporary* stability
> - Be constructed to allow computer tomography (CT) scanning of articular injuries
> - Allow all further treatment options
> - Achieve satisfactory indirect reduction
> - *And* mean that subsequent reconstruction is *easier and safer*

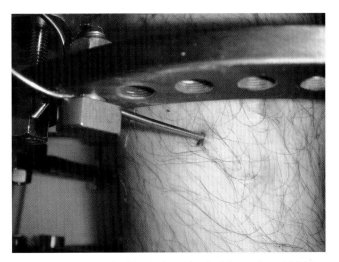

Figure 13.3 Pin site – a healthy pin site with only slight exudate which has dried.

became clear that certain groups of very severely injured patients were not able to tolerate the lengthy procedures needed for 'early total care' exemplified by femoral nailing. Alternative methods of spanning external fixation have been promoted in these circumstances. The goal is to provide the benefits of early fracture stabilization, without the risks of lengthy and often difficult surgery, carrying the risk of blood loss and bone marrow embolization. Once the patient has recovered sufficiently, then the temporary external fixator is exchanged for definitive surgery.

Similar techniques are also used for complex injuries such as fractures of the distal tibial articular surface (tibial plafond). Here the goal is to span the zone of injury, providing relative stability to the fracture, and achieve indirect reduction by using the frame to apply traction to the fracture fragments. The frame should be constructed in such a way that computed tomography (CT) scanning for the articular injury can be carried out easily.

Whether temporary or definitive, the frame should be applied in one of two ways. In the *frame first* technique the surgeon attaches the frame as two separate modules, one above and the other below the fracture. These are then used almost like handles to reduce the fracture and are then secured to each other. The other, less commonly employed method is the *reduction first* method. Here, as the name suggests, the limb is held reduced and the frame applied. This is much trickier than it sounds (Box 13.2).

Both threaded half-pins and fine wires can only be introduced via safe corridors, so their insertion carries the lowest risk of injuring nerves, blood vessels or tendons. Broadly speaking, each side of the fracture is secured with near–far fixation. This means a threaded half-pin, or wire, or both, near to the fracture, and the same again in a far position, thus gaining the most secure hold on a fracture fragment. There are some common sense limitations of this principle; for example, if a frame is applied to span a severe injury to the knee, then a very proximal pin in the thigh would stop the patient being able to sit up. A slightly more distal pin position is chosen.

With more complex frames for definitive care exemplified by Ilizarov circular frames, excellent reductions can be achieved and held with absolute stability, allowing weight-bearing in the frame. These frames are very versatile and can be used to carry out bone transport or bone lengthening to treat segmental defects.

Such frames can be in place for months or even years. Care of the pin sites is of paramount importance in the prevention of infection.

Pin care

Care of frames and pin sites hinges upon hygiene and is most effective if carried out by a well-motivated patient (Figures 13.3 and 13.4). Daily showers and cleaning the pin sites with simple soapy water and cotton buds while in the shower is best. The frame and limb can then be dried with a hairdryer. While the patient is in hospital, sterile gloves must always be used when dealing with pin sites and great care taken to avoid microbial cross-contamination, e.g. with methicillin-resistant *Staphylococcus aureus* (MRSA).

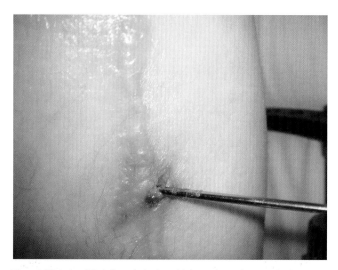

Figure 13.4 A mildly infected pin site which requires release under local anaesthetic.

Table 13.1 Troubleshooting pin sites.

Symptom	Action
Postoperative leakage	Leave undisturbed for 5 days Then clean with saline or in a shower
Skin tenting or tension	Skin release This may need to be repeated
Exudative pin site	Clean, release and repeat as required Dress with single thickness paraffin gauze
In-patients	Infection precautions at all times: • Dressings • Gloves
Infected pin site	Erythema and purulent discharge Clean, release, 5 days oral antibiotics

intra-articular fractures. Septic arthritis can occur which can be devastating, so these need close review.

Infection

Infection following fracture treatment, by either closed conservative or operative means is thankfully rare. When it does occur it can prove devastating. Wounds in certain areas and associated with surgery for particular fractures are prone to breakdown resulting from local soft tissue trauma, and the inherently poor blood supply of the tissue. Hence, these are at particular risk of infection. Such incisions include the distal part of the incision used to approach the anteromedial distal tibia, and also the incisions for calcaneal fractures.

Postoperative acute suppurative infections are rare, but easily recognized by the usual signs of acute inflammation, with a painful, red, hot, swollen surgical area. Provided there is no collection in the wound, antibiotics are usually sufficient. Any discharge that fails to resolve rapidly, or any obvious collection, must be evacuated in the operating theatre and the wound thoroughly cleaned. Repeated washouts are often required, supported by antibiotic treatment based upon fresh deep cultures from the wound. Removal of internal fixation can prove necessary along with conversion to an alternative form of fracture stabilization. Infected non-union of the fracture can result, which may then lead on to all the challenges associated with limb salvage surgery. Whole segments of unstable dead infected bone can be resected, with the limb supported in an Ilizarov frame. The bone void can then be reconstructed using a variety of methods ranging from free tissue transfer to bone transport.

Infections complicating fracture surgery are *always* serious, and can endanger the patient's limb, and their life.

Plaster

Plaster of Paris is applied to fractured limbs for two reasons. In the first instance, incomplete or backslab plasters are applied for rapid fracture immobilization and therefore pain relief. It is inhumane not to immobilize an obviously fractured limb in a backslab without a very good reason.

There are three phases to pin site care:

1 *Postoperative pin site care*: all pin sites will leak postoperatively. Leave them undisturbed for 5 days, then take down the dressings and clean the pin sites, either in the shower (if the patient is well enough) or with normal saline and cotton buds. *All* blood clot and granulation must be cleared. If the skin is tented or under tension from the wire, a release can be performed. Wires that have been released or show signs of having crusted with scab or exudates should be dressed with a small single-thickness square of paraffin gauze and dressing gauze. The smaller the better.

2 *The exudative pin site*: because swelling will come and go after surgery and as the patient starts to mobilize, pin sites often crust up with clot or clear exudates. Thorough cleaning needs to be followed by a release performed under local anaesthetic, which may need to be repeated several times as the weeks go by and the skin finds its own best position beside the wire. This is most common at the ankle and knee, as the skin there is the most mobile. Again, apply a small single-thickness square of paraffin gauze and dressing gauze afterwards. The patient should not then shower for 48 hours, just to let things settle. All pin sites in in-patients must be dressed. The rate of MRSA colonization is high, and this is acquired in hospital.

3 *The epithelialized pin site*: all pin sites should eventually epithelialize right up to the wire. These can then be left open to the air, but with the frame covered in a Tubigrip to keep off unwanted visitors such as dogs and flies.

All patients should have a night splint made (by the plaster room) to stop the foot falling into equinus (foot drop). This can be carried out on day 1 or 2 postoperatively. Physiotherapy to assist weight-bearing and avoid knee and ankle contractures is essential.

Occasionally, pin sites become actively infected, and have a flare of erythema and purulent discharge (Table 13.1). This normally settles with a clean, a release and 5 days of oral antibiotics. Extra care should be taken with infection of wires close to the knee in

Table 13.2 Troubleshooting plaster of Paris. Replacing a cast in an unstable fracture runs the risk of re-displacement. This must be checked with radiographs after the new well-molded cast is applied. If the fracture requires reduction again this must be attended to promptly.

Symptom	Action
Increasing pain	Split cast and wool padding to the skin: • Pain relief should be immediate • Beware compartment syndrome
Pressure areas	Ensure adequate padding over bony prominences
Loose fitting	Remove and apply a new cast
Wet/smelly	Remove and apply a new cast
Cast broken, degenerating	Remove and apply a new cast

Plaster of Paris casts can also be used very successfully to maintain fracture reduction, and are commonly used in children's fractures. Injured limbs will swell more, even after immobilization, and so increasing pain in a cast is an absolute indication to split the cast and cotton wool padding all the way down to the skin and prize that cast apart a little. The relief from this intervention should be almost instantaneous. If is not, the patient may well be developing compartment syndrome (see below).

The other main problems associated with plasters relate to pressure problems on the skin, and stiffness in adjacent joints (Table 13.2). Great care must be taken in cast application to ensure adequate padding of bony prominences and also the ends of the cast to prevent rubbing. When plastering above the elbow, it is important to avoid excessive padding in the antecubital fossa and the crook of the elbow. This can act like a tourniquet.

Another common error is to extend the cast too far over the palm restricting finger movement. This is especially important in the elderly, in whom permanent stiffness can develop quite rapidly.

Compartment syndrome

Compartment syndrome occurs when the tissue pressure in a compartment exceeds the tissue perfusion pressure at a capillary level, and muscle and nerve ischaemia occurs. Left untreated, the best that can be hoped for is ischaemic contracture of the muscles as they fibrose, leading to deformity and a useless limb. Worse still, crush syndrome may supervene, with myoglobin and potassium being liberated from the damaged muscle. Acute hyperkalaemia can be lethal, and renal failure from myoglobinuria can be permanent. The only effective treatment for compartment syndrome is fasciotomy.

Recognition of compartment syndrome hinges upon suspicion. Mechanism of injury is a major factor in the development of this complication. It is also relatively common after intramedullary nailing of tibial fractures. The presentation of compartment syndrome is radically different depending upon whether the patient is awake or not.

The conscious patient will do everything in their power to tell the nursing and medical staff that something is wrong. Their pain worsens despite analgesia, and examination will reveal a patient in great distress. Skin capillary perfusion and peripheral pulses are almost always completely normal, unless the compartment syndrome is also associated with a major vascular injury. Any nerve passing deep through the affected compartment will be ischaemic. Thus, with compartment syndrome of the lower limb, the first web space on the foot (the cutaneous distribution of the deep branch of the common peroneal nerve) will have diminished or even absent sensation when compared to the opposite limb. There will be virtually no active movement in the digits and passive movement causes extreme pain. In such circumstances, the diagnosis is made and pressure measurements are not necessary.

The unconscious patient, or someone post nerve block, poses a greater diagnostic problem. Suspicion, vigilance and early (and sometime repeated) measurement of the compartment pressures are essential. If the compartment pressure is within 30 mmHg of the diastolic blood pressure, the diagnosis is confirmed and fasciotomy is indicated.

Fasciotomy rescues muscle from irretrievable ischaemia and also allows débridement of dead tissue. This may need to be repeated several times and closure may require split skin grafting.

Remember, only walk away from the patient to take to theatre immediately, or with certainty that there is no compartment syndrome. *If there is any doubt there is no doubt.*

Fasciotomy wounds may be closed after the swelling has settled, either primarily with sutures or by serial tightening of 'lacing' attached to the skin edges. If primary closure is not possible, then the epithelialized muscle will need to be skin grafted.

Further reading

Stannard JP, Schmidt AH, Kregor PJ. *Surgical Treatment of Orthopaedic Trauma.* Thieme, New York, 2007.

Index